Ask the Vet

ABOUT CATS

Easy Answers to Commonly Asked Questions

D1406889

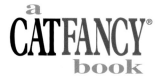

a
CATFANCY®
book

by Elaine Wexler-Mitchell, D.V.M.

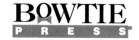

BOWTIE
PRESS®

A DIVISION OF BOWTIE, INC.
IRVINE, CALIFORNIA

Jen Dorsey, Project Manager
Nick Clemente, Special Consultant
Karla Austin, Business Operations Manager
Michelle Martinez, Assistant Editor
Book design by Michele Lanci-Altomare
Layout by Michael Vincent Capozzi

Library of Congress Cataloging-in-Publication Data

Wexler-Mitchell, Elaine.
  Ask the vet : easy answers to commonly asked questions / by Elaine
Wexler-Mitchell.
      p. cm.
"A cat fancy book."
  ISBN 1-931993-00-9 (pbk. : alk. paper)
  1. Cats—Miscellanea. 2. Cats—Health—Miscellanea. I. Title.

SF447 .W478 2003
636.8—dc21

                                    2002014280

BowTie Press®
A Division of BowTie, Inc.
3 Burroughs
Irvine, California 92618

Printed and Bound in Singapore
10 9 8 7 6 5 4 3 2 1

Contents

Introduction 7

■ Behavior 9
How do I prevent my cat from scratching furniture? 10
How do I stop my cat from biting? 11
How can I stop my cat from chewing on things? 11
How can I tell if my cat grooms excessively, and what can I do to prevent
    this? 12
How do I train my cat to use a litter box? 13
My cat started urinating outside the litter box. What can I do? 13
Why does my cat spray, and how do I stop her from spraying? 15
How do I introduce a new cat in the household if I already have a cat? . . . 16
My cat hides from me. What can I do? 17
How can I keep my cat from freaking out when I take her to the vet? 17
My cat meows constantly. Is there anything I can do? 18
How do I keep my cat from eating or destroying my plants? 19

■ Diet and Digestion 21
Is dry cat food better than canned for my cat's teeth and gums? 22
What does it mean if my cat stops eating? 22
How can I stop my cat's frequent vomiting? 23
How can I firm up my cat's stool? 23
How do I know if my cat is constipated? What can I do? 24
What can I do to help my cat with hairballs? 25
My cat likes to play with strings. Is this dangerous? 25
My cat goes outside and likes to hunt. Is this dangerous? 26
What does it mean if my cat becomes jaundiced? 26
How do I know if my cat is at a healthy weight? 27

■ Parasites and Zoonoses 29
How do I know if my cat has worms? 30

Can I get parasites from my cat? 31
What other parasites can cause gastrointestinal disease? 31
What methods of flea control work best? 32
How do I know if my cat has mange? 33
Can I get ringworm from my cat? 33
If I'm pregnant, can I handle my cat? 34
What is cat scratch disease? 34
Can my cat get Lyme disease? 35
Is my cat at risk for heartworms? 35
My cat has flea allergy dermatitis. What can I do to make my cat more
    comfortable? 36
Why does my kitten still have loose stool after testing negative for
    parasites? 36
If my cat scratches her ears, does she have ear mites? 37

■ Vaccines and Routine Care 39
How do I administer medicine to my cat? 40
Should I vaccinate my cat? If so, how often? 41
What is the FRCP vaccine? 42
What are feline leukemia and feline AIDS? 43
How can my cat contract rabies? 44
How will I know if my cat is having a reaction to a vaccine? 45
What other vaccines are there? 46
When will my kitten lose his baby teeth? 47
What happens when a cat is declawed? 48
What form of identification will help my cat get found if he gets lost? 48
Can routine vaccines cause cancer? 49

■ First Aid and Emergency Care 51
How do I find an emergency animal clinic? 52
How can I tell if my cat has a fever? 52
Is it safe to give my cat aspirin? 53
What should I do if my cat gets into a fight? 54
What should I do if I cut a toenail too short and it bleeds? 55

What should I do if my cat gets overheated? 55

What should I do if I suspect my cat has fractured a limb? 56

How dangerous is antifreeze to cats? 56

What should I do if my cat eats something that's bad for her? 57

What should I do if a bee or wasp stings my cat? 58

What should I do if my cat is hit by a car? 58

What does it mean if there is blood in my cat's stool? 59

My cat is rapidly losing weight. What can this mean? 59

■ Reproduction 61

At what age can I sterilize my pet? 62

Should I let my female cat go through a heat cycle before I spay her? 63

Why should I neuter my male cat? 64

How long is a cat pregnant? 64

Can my cat get pregnant while she is nursing a litter? 65

What can be done to stop an accidental pregnancy? 65

At what age should I wean my kitten? 65

My male cat only has one testicle. Should I be concerned? 66

What should I do about my cat's vaginal discharge? 67

Should I be concerned about a lump in my cat's mammary region? 67

Is there anything I can do to help control the stray cat population? 68

Is herpes transferable from a mother cat to her kittens? 68

I am interested in breeding my cat, but I am concerned about hip dysplasia.
    Is it hereditary? 69

■ Geriatrics 71

How do I calculate the age of my cat in human years? When is a cat old? . 72

When is my cat too old to handle anesthesia? 72

Can my cat eat if she is missing teeth? 73

What does it mean if my cat drinks excessive amounts of water? 74

Can cats have high blood pressure? 74

What happens to a cat with hyperthyroidism? 75

How can I tell if my cat has cancer? 75

Do cats get arthritis? 76

How is heart disease diagnosed in cats? 77

How do I know when it is time to put my cat to sleep? 78

My cat has diabetes mellitus. What care do I need to provide her? 79

General Health 81

What are some general ways I can help protect my cat from disease? 82

Should I have my cat's teeth cleaned? 82

How can I tell if my cat can't see? 83

What can I do if my cat's eye is red and squinting? 84

Can cats develop allergies? 84

Can I catch a cold from my cat? 85

What should I do if my cat is straining to urinate? 86

What should I do if my cat gags and wheezes? 87

My cat's coat doesn't look good. Could there be a problem? 88

I would like to take my cat on vacation with me.

     What steps should I take to prepare him for a trip? 88

Should I get pet insurance? 89

My cat is shaking his head and scratching his ears.

     What, besides ear mites, can cause this? 90

What can I do to prevent impacted anal glands? 90

Should I worry if my cat pants excessively? 90

How often should I take my cat to the veterinarian? 91

How do I deal with the death of my cat? 91

Conclusion 92

Index 93

Introduction

I have practiced small animal veterinary medicine for the past seventeen years and started my own practice exclusive to felines in 1991. In working in everyday clinical practice over the years, I've had the opportunity to interact with thousands of clients and their cats, and have learned what questions people commonly ask regarding the care and husbandry of their cats. I have also written for *Cat Fancy* magazine's "Ask the Vet" column. In doing so, I've read thousands of reader inquiry letters and e-mails regarding feline care. I hope that by drawing from these experiences I can help you give your cats the best care possible by answering some of the most commonly asked feline questions. The questions addressed in this book range from basic knowledge to specific problems that cat owners can be faced with everyday.

This book is not meant to replace veterinary care but to give you the background information you need to care for your cat. A good relationship with a competent veterinarian is essential in maintaining a healthy cat. I hope that you will find the information in this book useful and easy to reference throughout your years of cat ownership.

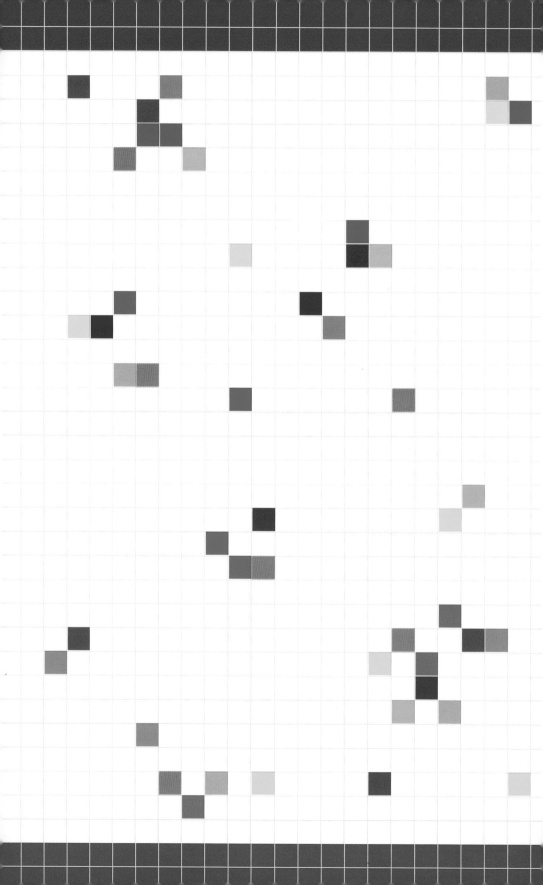

CHAPTER 1

Behavior

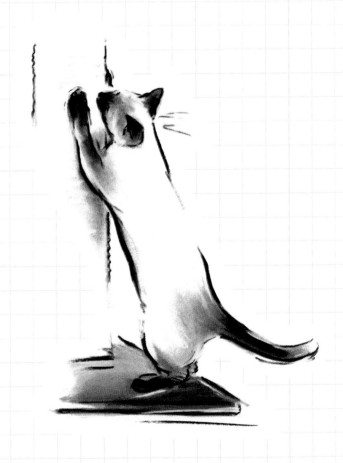

Cats are distinctive pets in that their independent nature often outweighs their desire to please their owners. Cats have temperaments and genetics that result in behavior issues that are unique to the species. Behavior issues that make a cat owner lose sleep may not even cross the mind of a dog owner. For example, the way cats groom and eliminate is vastly different from that of dogs. A trip to the vet may be a fun car ride for a dog, but it can be extremely upsetting for a cat. Behavior problems are serious and can often affect the long-term relationship you will have with your cat. If you can catch pesky problems early and work together with your cat to modify her behavior, your relationship can be rewarding instead of taxing. Keep in mind that you as owner are ultimately responsible—your cat deserves your full attention at all times, especially when it comes to behavior issues.

Q *How do I prevent my cat from scratching furniture?*

A Scratching is a normal behavior for a cat. Scratching keeps a cat's nails in shape and leaves her scent on the area she scratches. Some cats prefer to scratch carpet, while others prefer sisal (high fiber twine). Some like vertical posts and others horizontal corrugated cardboard. Unless you train your cat, she will not know the difference between a scratching post and a sofa or carpet.

To train your cat to use a scratching post, make it part of her morning routine, even before feeding, by encouraging her over to the post by dangling a toy. Cats follow habitual patterns of behavior, and this should establish a routine. If you have a kitten, introduce her to scratching posts early on. If your cat has already started scratching an off-limits item, you need to break the habit as soon as possible. Squirting her with water, covering the item with a plastic drop cloth, or applying double sided tape to the item are some options. Another option that works with some cats is repellant spray; many cats stop scratching items that have been sprayed with Feliway, a spray that is a chemical copy of feline facial pheromones.

Also, try placing a scratching post next to the item you don't want scratched and move the cat over to it when the cat is scratching the wrong item or during play. Once the cat has started using the post, move it to a more desirable location a few feet at a time over the course of a week.

Q How do I stop my cat from biting?

A Cats bite during play, if they are startled or injured, and if they are aggressive. When a kitten is small she seems fun and harmless when she nibbles or attacks your hand, but if not prevented, this behavior will continue as she gets older. While adults can usually physically handle this type of biting, small children cannot and often become scared of the cat. Either way, if you have guests at your home, they may not appreciate their hands being bitten, since your kitty thinks of any hand as a toy.

The best way to prevent biting is by never allowing your cat to bite any part of your body. You should have one or two toys that are delegated as bite toys. Cats like to bite soft things. A stuffed sock or stuffed animals are good substitutions for your hands and feet. Use these objects to play with your cat or put in your cat's mouth when she starts to bite.

Despite giving cats something appropriate to bite, they sometimes still get wild and out of control. If this occurs, a "kitty time-out" is in order and can be achieved by closing your cat into a small room (with or without lights) by herself for ten to fifteen minutes. During this period, your cat can calm down and then be reintroduced to your home. If the biting behavior starts again, put your kitty back into isolation. If a cat bites in an unpredictable manner, consider carrying a squirt gun and squirting her when she bites, avoiding her eyes and face. Cat bites are dangerous because of the likelihood of infection, so if you cannot control your cat's biting seek professional guidance from your veterinarian.

Q How can I stop my cat from chewing on things?

A Some cats chew on objects to get attention, and others just develop the bad habit. Chewing on items such as electrical cords is dangerous, as is the ingestion of objects that can lodge in the intestine and cause obstructions.

If you discover that your cat has a desire to chew on certain items, you need to place these items out of your cat's reach when possible. If your cat compulsively chews, try to retrain her by offering appropriate chew items and making inappropriate objects taste bad. If the items are accessible to your cat, spray a bad-tasting substance such as Bitter Apple or Yuck gel on the items to discourage chewing. Toys (with or without catnip), cat grass, and rawhide chews are some appropriate chew items you can use to train your cat. If your cat is attracted to electrical wires or phone cords, place them inside stiff PVC pipes to hide them. If training is unsuccessful, your vet may recommend oral treatment with antianxiety medications.

Q *How can I tell if my cat grooms excessively, and what can I do to prevent this?*

A You can tell that your cat grooms excessively if she makes herself bald or red in certain areas of her skin or creates open sores. Cats normally groom about one-third of the time that they are not sleeping, but this does not usually cause any irritation or noticeable hair loss. Veterinarians call excessive grooming psychogenic alopecia if it is a behavioral reaction to stress. The condition is similar to that of humans who bite their fingernails too low—it's an unconscious habit. Your veterinarian should eliminate medical causes for excessive grooming such as fleas, allergies, or bacterial or fungal infections before he or she can diagnose psychogenic alopecia.

Cats who overgroom tend to vomit more hairballs than average cats due to the ingestion of extra hair. Some cats overgroom because they are bored or want to attract their owner's attention. If your cat grooms excessively but doesn't create bald patches or more extensive lesions, try to interrupt the behavior and engage her in another activity such as petting or play. If bald areas or sores exist, the temporary use of an Elizabethan collar, a lampshade-like protective collar that prevents the cat from grooming or chewing on herself, can help to break the behavior problem and gives the skin time to heal. Bad-tasting topical sprays are also useful for discouraging the constant licking. Antihistamines, herbal calming remedies, and antianxiety medications can all be used to break the cycle and calm your cat. See your veterinarian for a recommendation specific to your cat.

Q *How do I train my cat to use a litter box?*

A Eliminating in a litter box is a natural behavior for cats. To reinforce this behavior, place the litter box in an area easily accessible to your cat and fill with plain litter (litter that is unscented). Place your cat gently in the box. To stimulate digging, place your hand on your cat's paw and make the same motion she would if she were digging. Let your cat sniff and explore the box.

Introducing your cat to the litter box should be adequate enough for her to begin using the box regularly. You should, however, monitor the box for use—most cats urinate twice daily and defecate once daily—to be sure your cat is using the litter box. Keep the box clean by scooping it at least once daily. If your cat has an accident outside the box, never yell at her and throw her into the litter box. Doing so creates fear of the litter box and causes a litter box aversion. It is best to keep one litter box per cat. Two cats, however, can share one box as long as it is kept clean and is large enough to accommodate them.

Q *My cat started urinating outside the litter box. What can I do?*

A Urinating outside the litter box and spraying are two different problems. Cats direct inappropriate elimination outside the litter box onto horizontal surfaces, such as the floor, not onto vertical surfaces as in spraying. Inappropriate elimination is either caused by urinary tract disease or behavioral problems. Behavioral problems that may cause inappropriate elimination are difficult to determine because situations that create stress or anxiety for your cat may not be apparent to you.

Make sure that you are keeping your cat's litter box as clean as possible by scooping it twice daily. If you changed the type of litter you use in the litter box, your cat may not like it; cats have preferences for certain types of litter. If there are no obvious litter box factors, have your cat examined and her urine analyzed. If urinalysis and examination uncover a medical problem, your veterinarian will make treatment recommendations.

If there are no obvious medical problems, you need to work with your veterinarian or a behaviorist to identify the factors triggering the inappropriate elimination behavior. As with other behavior problems, the best chance for stopping inappropriate elimination is with early intervention. It is unrealistic to think that a behavior pattern that has been in existence for more than a couple of weeks can be turned around within a few days, so be patient and compliant with your vet's recommendation. You will achieve the best results with a combination of behavior modification and antianxiety drug therapy. Give your cat plenty of attention and set aside at least five minutes twice a day to play with your cat to decrease stress and boredom and create a new behavior pattern.

You will need to clean and neutralize areas of elimination so that your cat is not attracted back to the same spot. Avoid cleaners with ammonia as they intensify the smell of urine and make your cat want to eliminate in the same area. In addition to cleaners, you can create an obstruction or spray a repellant on the affected area. To create an obstruction, simply close the door to the affected room, place an additional litter box on the area, put a plastic carpet runner placed upside down on the area, lay down aluminum foil, or play with and feed your cat at the site. Repel your cat from affected areas using solid air fresheners with a fruity or flowery scent. Cats do not like fruity or flowery scents; they only like their own. There are numerous brands available in grocery and drug stores.

If these steps are not successful, you can also use herbal calming remedies and antianxiety medications along with behavior modification to treat inappropriate elimination caused by behavioral problems. Some of the prescription drugs used are amitriptyline (Elavil), clomipramine

(Clomicalm), buspirone (BusPar), paroxetine (Paxil), and fluoxetine hydrochloride (Prozac). Some cats can be weaned off the medication eventually, but others need long-term treatment to keep their behavior under control. You should avoid hormone therapy for inappropriate elimination due to the potential for side effects, such diabetes mellitus or mammary cancer. Curing an inappropriate elimination problem requires early recognition, owner commitment, and patience.

Q *Why does my cat spray, and how do I stop her from spraying?*

A Spraying (squirting urine onto a vertical surface such as a door or wall) is a territorial behavior, usually triggered when a cat feels threatened by another cat. Cats tend to spray doors and windows because this is where other cats can be seen or heard. Cats also spray when their litter box is dirty or when they have urinary tract problems. Both male and female cats can spray.

Spaying or neutering your cat before she or he reaches puberty (six to eight months of age) is the best preventive measure against spraying. Also, simply being aware of your cat's whereabouts and spraying tendencies will help. Since cats tend to spray the same surfaces repeatedly because they smell the scent of their urine, you should clean sprayed surfaces with an enzyme cleaner designed for cat odors as soon as you discover the sprayed area. After the cleaned area is dry, you can apply Feliway, which contains a feline facial pheromone. Pheromones are chemical messengers that trigger behaviors, and the pheromone produced by cells in the cheek area triggers a friendly response that makes most cats feel relaxed and nonthreatened so they will be less likely to spray. When possible, keep your cat out of rooms where other cats can be seen or heard. Consider placing cat repellant around the perimeter of your home to keep other cats away.

If your cat's spraying behavior continues, consult your veterinarian to determine whether an underlying medical problem exists or if antianxiety medication is an option. Avoid treating your cat with hormones to prevent spraying; they have the potential for serious side effects, such as diabetes mellitus and mammary cancer.

Q *How do I introduce a new cat in the household if I already have a cat?*

A It is best to bring a new cat into your household because you want to have another pet, not because you think your cat needs a companion. Introducing a new cat can pose a challenge because not all cats are compatible. It is usually easier to introduce a young cat into a home that has an older cat because a young cat will not initially be territorial or threaten the status of the existing cat. Cats of the opposite sex will not necessarily get along better than cats of the same sex. The issue of compatibility comes down to individual cat personalities and chemistry. In some situations, it takes months for cats to adjust to each other, although sometimes they never become friends and simply cohabitate.

When introducing your cat to a new cat, avoid making your cat feel like her territory is being invaded by slowly acquainting the cats. Isolate the new cat to a closed-off room for a week with her own food, water, and litter box and observe her for sneezing, runny eyes, vomiting, and diarrhea. Isolation helps to prevent the spreading of any infectious diseases from the new cat to your cat and also allows your cat an opportunity to get used to having another cat in the home.

Ideally, any new cat should be examined by a veterinarian and given a clean bill of health. When you are sure that the new cat is in good health, the next step is a supervised introduction. Place the new cat in a carrier and have your cat inspect the carrier. Another option is to hold the new cat and bring her into a room with your cat and see what their responses are. It is normal for cats to hiss at each other initially but rare for them to be physically aggressive. Increase the amount of time the cats spend together until you feel comfortable having them together unsupervised.

Q *My cat hides from me. What can I do?*

A Cats have personalities that differ from one cat to another, making some cats more loving and social than others. Their personalities are based on genetics and their environment during the critical socialization period of two to seven weeks of age. If cats do not favorably bond with humans during socialization, they are fearful of people, and it is more difficult for them to be affectionate later in life. Fearfulness causes cats to hide, but this doesn't mean that they have been harmed or treated badly in the past. It only means that they haven't received loving human contact during the socialization period.

You can change your cat's tentative behavior with positive reinforcement. The key is finding a treat or toy that especially appeals to your cat and using it as a training tool to motivate your cat. Use this treat to reward your cat when she lets you pet her. Some people think that smothering a cat with attention is more effective than slowly gaining trust and acceptance. You may need to try both approaches and see how your cat responds. Work with rewarding your cat in a quiet, nonthreatening environment. It can take months to change any behavior problem in your cat, so be patient and keep trying. If you allow your cat to hide and make no attempt to change her behavior, it is unlikely that the situation will change.

Q *How can I keep my cat from freaking out when I take her to the vet?*

A Cats are in tune with their owners' body language. So, if you feel anxious when you take your cat to the vet, your cat will probably feel anxious, too. Your cat may also feel stress when she knows she has to enter her carrier, which means the veterinary visit is already off to a bad start. But there are a few tricks you can use to help minimize your cat's stress.

Remain calm when taking your cat to the vet. This will help reduce your cat's anxiety. If you have difficulty getting your cat into a carrier, try leaving the carrier out and open for a day or two before the vet visit or consider buying another type of carrier, such as one that opens at the end and from the top and has quick release hinges that makes it easy to use. You can also try putting her into a pillowcase, then into the carrier. Sometimes if a cat is covered up she is calmer because she thinks she is hiding.

Despite following the steps above, your cat may still get anxious and defensive. Administering an herbal calming remedy or a prescription tranquilizer an hour or two before a visit helps reduce anxiety. If you suspect that your cat is not going to behave well in the veterinary office, it is best to alert the staff before they begin to handle your cat so that no one gets hurt or exacerbates the situation. Unfortunately, your cat may still get scared and aggressive and your veterinarian may suggest an injectable sedation. Sedation may be the best alternative for allowing a safe and thorough examination or treatment of a cat.

Q *My cat meows constantly. Is there anything I can do?*

A Cats meow for a variety of reasons, but it is usually because they want or need something from you. Your cat may want to go outside to explore the neighborhood. She may be hungry. Or, she may want to sit in your favorite chair. Geriatric cats meow if they become disoriented or if they have problems such as high blood pressure. The reasons cats meow are as diverse as the animals themselves.

Some cats meow more than others. Certain breeds like Siamese and Oriental Shorthairs are ingrained with a tendency to make a lot of noise. If you own one of these breeds, you may have no choice but to tune out the chatter from your cat.

Many cats meow more than others because they have learned that vocalizing their needs is the easiest way to get their owners to acquiesce. Every time you answer your cat's call by giving her food, letting her outside, or fetching her favorite toy, you reinforce her behavior. To help curb her "talking," you can try spraying water (avoiding the eyes and face) or shaking a can of pennies in her direction and not giving in to her demands. Be consistent with breaking her cycle of meowing and you will see results sooner rather than later.

Q *How do I keep my cat from eating or destroying my plants?*

A Cats tend to chew plant leaves, probably as a way to ingest natural fiber in their diets. Be aware that not all plants are safe for your cat to eat, and no plant is safe if it has been treated with chemicals. Some of the more common plants that are unsafe for your cat are aloe vera, calla lily, several kinds of ivy, philodendron, tomato plant, and tulip. Check with your veterinarian or the National Animal Poison Control Center for a complete list of toxic plants. Some plants, like catnip, parsley, and thyme are kitty safe, so you might want to pot some indoors or plant them in your herb garden so your cat has a safe nibbling alternative.

The dirt in your potted plants may appeal to your cat as an appropriate place to urinate or defecate, since in the wild, or if left outdoors, cats naturally eliminate in dirt or sand. Your cat may simply think the potted plant is just another litter box.

Keep plants safe from cats (and vice versa) by relocating some of your more prized plants to higher ground by putting them on high shelves or hanging them. If plants must stay on the floor or lower tables and shelves, you can spray the plant's leaves with Bitter Apple spray so they taste bad to prevent chewing or rub leaves with ginger powder—it has a bitter taste. Garden stores sell safe products that can be placed in soil to deter pets from plants.

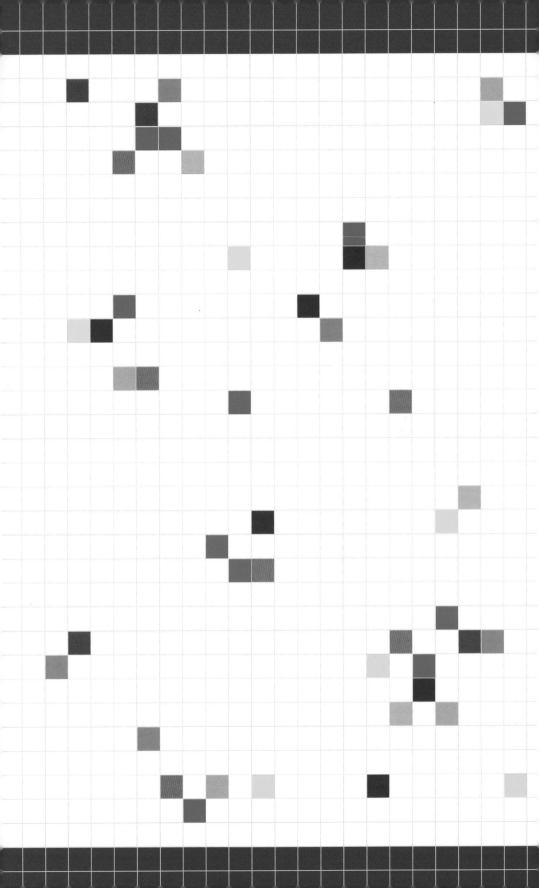

CHAPTER 2

Diet and Digestion

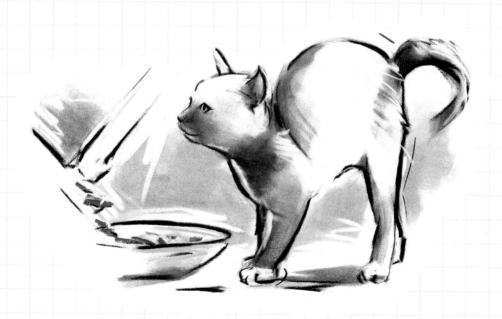

One might think that feeding a cat is a simple task that requires little thought. Actually, cats—like humans—require certain essential nutrients for good health. Consider that what you feed your cat affects several different parts of his body such as teeth, gums, intestine, bowel, and even skin and coat. Choosing the right food for your cat is an important decision. Likewise, monitoring weight and hairball production are important factors in your cat's overall digestive health.

Q **Is dry cat food better than canned for my cat's teeth and gums?**

A Dry cat food is better for your cat's teeth and gums because it doesn't stick to the teeth as much as canned, which can lead to plaque and tartar buildup. Also there are dry food products specifically formulated for your cat's dental health. These products create an abrasive action on the teeth when chewed and contain ingredients that decrease the formation of plaque. Though dry food is better for your cat's teeth it is not necessarily better for his general health; most nutritionists think a combination is best.

Even if your cat exclusively eats dry cat food, plaque and tartar can build on the teeth from a combination of food and saliva, so proper dental hygiene is important. Good dental health results from a combination of diet, home dental care, and professional dental care through your veterinarian.

Q **What does it mean if my cat stops eating?**

A Cats stop eating for a variety of reasons, including an unappetizing diet, dental disease, fever, loss of smell, and stress. Your cat can be in danger if he does not eat for an extended period of time. When your cat does not eat, the fat his body has stored is metabolized to provide energy. Too much fat breakdown damages the liver and leads to another condition called hepatic lipidosis, also known as fatty liver disease.

To tempt your cat to eat, try warming some baby food. Warm food generates an appetizing smell, which should encourage your cat to eat, and baby food is easy for your cat to digest. If your cat does not eat for two days, a veterinarian should examine him as soon as possible.

Q How can I stop my cat's frequent vomiting?

A A healthy cat can experience frequent vomiting. Causes range from food intolerance, eating too quickly, ingesting plants or paper, playing too hard after eating, and ingesting hairballs to medical conditions such as early inflammatory bowel disease. You need to observe vomiting episodes, taking note of contents, frequency, time of day, association with eating, and general health of the cat to help determine the cause. These observations will aid your veterinarian in reaching a diagnosis.

Cats who vomit within a few minutes of eating are actually regurgitating and need to slow down when they eat. To decrease regurgitation, try one the following: mix canned and dry food together (cats cannot eat the combination as quickly); add water to dry kibble, so the pieces expand, before letting your cat eat it (the food will not expand in the stomach and create overfilling); feed your cat larger kibble that requires chewing; put food in a shallower bowl so the food is thinly dispersed and cannot be ingested in large mouthfuls; feed multiple cats separately to decrease competition; and feed smaller and more frequent meals. You should discuss ongoing vomiting and/or regurgitation with your veterinarian.

Q How can I firm up my cat's stool?

A Cats normally have firm, formed stool. Soft stool results from intestinal parasites, food intolerance, dietary indiscretion (eating things your cat shouldn't), inadequate fiber intake, stress, and disease such as colitis. Many owners feed their cats a variety of foods, treats, and table scraps. Although your cat may enjoy eating these items, they are not equally well digested thus lead to variations in stool. Cats who go outside may ingest food they hunt or eat another cat's food at a neighbor's home, which may also cause soft stool.

If you are unable to identify food items that trigger soft stools, and you cannot control stool consistency with one particular diet, you can try giving your cat a pet psyllium fiber supplement such as Vetasyl. If stools are still soft, ask your vet to check your cat for intestinal parasites and other health problems.

Q *How do I know if my cat is constipated? What can I do?*

A A cat can become constipated because of inadequate water intake, poor diet, lack of fiber, too much hair in the stool, general inactivity, and intestinal muscle dysfunction. Cats who don't eat don't produce stool, which can be confused with constipation. Be sure to rule this out before administering a remedy for constipation. One way to tell the difference is that cats with constipation strain when they try to defecate, it is not that they simply don't defecate.

It is important for you to observe your cat when he visits the litter box frequently to determine whether he is having difficulty defecating or urinating. Owners sometimes have difficulty distinguishing between the postures for urinating and defecating. Although constipation is an uncomfortable problem for a cat, an inability to urinate can turn into a life threatening condition for a male cat, so it is important for owners to recognize these postural differences. Cats typically defecate one to two times a day. If your cat does not have a bowel movement for two or more days, constipation is a possibility.

Two remedies that aid in relieving constipation are hairball lubricant pastes (they are also laxatives) and psyllium fiber supplements (fiber helps stimulate stool passage). These can be administered to your cat by following the printed directions and can be used until your cat is having regular bowel movements. If, after a day of unsuccessful home care, you are unable to relieve your cat's constipation or if constipation is an ongoing problem, consult with your veterinarian. Never give your cat an enema unless prescribed by a veterinarian, as some over-the-counter enemas contain phosphate, which is toxic to cats.

Q *What can I do to help my cat with hairballs?*

A Ingesting hairballs is normal for cats. Hairballs are created when hair that a cat ingests through grooming accumulates in the stomach or the intestines. The cat must pass this hair through his system either by vomiting or defecating to prevent an intestinal obstruction. There are hairball remedies available over-the-counter that you can administer to your cat to ensure that hairballs pass through a cat's system through vomiting or defecating.

Hairball remedies are designed to decrease the frequent vomiting of hairballs, but hairballs cannot be completely eliminated. Hairball remedies include pastes, chewable treats, fiber supplements, and specially formulated diets. You can choose between these options based on your cat's preference and response to treatment. Combing and brushing your cat thoroughly at least once weekly also decreases the amount of hair he ingests during self-grooming. Some owners have their cats shaved to reduce hair intake.

Q *My cat likes to play with strings. Is this dangerous?*

A Cats love to play with strings, ribbons, newspaper ties, yarn, dental floss, thread, and fishing line; but all of these items pose a danger to a cat if ingested. For no known reason, cats swallow these items, now called linear foreign bodies, when given the opportunity. Short pieces of linear objects can pass through a cat's intestinal tract but larger lengths get trapped and cause the intestines to bunch up, similar to a drawstring in a waistband. Left untreated, a linear foreign body leads to intestinal perforation and peritonitis, life threatening conditions that even with intensive care may not be treatable. It is safe for you and your cat to play with the above-mentioned items, but be sure to put them away when you can-not supervise playtime to prevent accidental ingestion.

Q *My cat goes outside and likes to hunt. Is this dangerous?*

A Hunting is a natural instinct for a cat. Cats stalk bugs, mice, rats, and birds. Some cats are satisfied with the thrill of the hunt, others kill and eat their prey. Many cats like to bring their prey home and present it to you. It is always a good idea to check your cat's mouth before letting him in the house. If a cat eats an animal who is sick with a viral or bacterial infection, or one who has been exposed to poisons such as rodenticides, he could be in danger. Bugs are also harmful as they can release or con-tain irritant chemicals that can cause nausea and drooling in cats. If your cat is a hunter and exhibits any clinical signs of illness, a veterinarian should examine him.

If your cat ventures outside, it is impossible to prevent hunting, even in a controlled environment such as a fenced-in yard. To warn potential prey that their stalker is nearby, attach a bell to your cat's col-lar; this should scare prey away but still give your cat the excitement of the hunt.

Q *What does it mean if my cat becomes jaundiced?*

A Jaundice is the yellowing of the skin, whites of the eyes, and gums. The yellowing occurs because pigments called bilirubin are released into the blood during the metabolic breakdown of hemoglobin, a component of red blood cells. This process occurs in the liver, which means jaundice is associated with a dysfunctional liver. Cats who are clinically jaundiced also produce bright orange urine (bilirubinuria).

A jaundiced cat should receive immediate medical attention, so contact your veterinarian immediately. Blood and urine tests help to determine the cause of the problem, but most often, the specific cause of liver disease cannot be diagnosed without a liver biopsy. Your veterinarian will perform a biopsy using a needle guided by ultrasound or through surgery. A veterinarian determines the extent of treatment and testing needed based on examination of the cat and clinical data. Most types of liver disease are treatable, since the liver is an organ able to regenerate itself.

Q *How do I know if my cat is at a healthy weight?*

A To determine whether your cat is at a healthy weight, pinch the skin over the ribs. If you clearly see your cat's ribs, he is too thin. If you pinch more than an inch, he is too heavy. Owners often mistake fatty areas in their cat's lower abdominal region (inguinal fat pads), as a sign of being overweight, but these are common in most adult cats. Cats in good body condition have a noticeable waist, but a bulging abdomen means your cat is overweight.

Getting a cat to lose weight is not easy. Tips for dieting include limiting food portions to amounts recommended on the package for a desired weight, feeding a diet lower in calories than the current diet, and exercising your cat through active play. Your veterinarian should monitor your cat's weight at least once a year.

If your cat is too thin, it could be a sign of more serious problems, like kidney disease. Consult your veterinarian if you suspect uncommon weight loss.

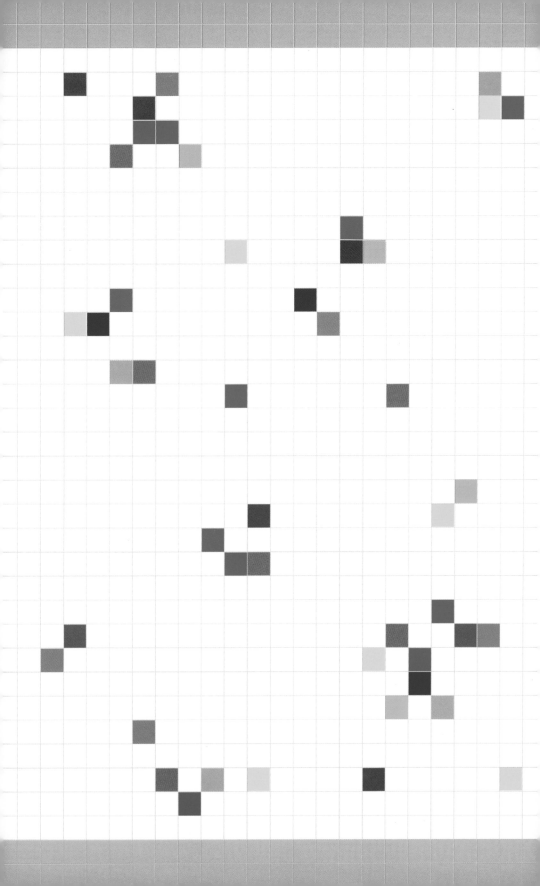

CHAPTER 3

Parasites and Zoonoses

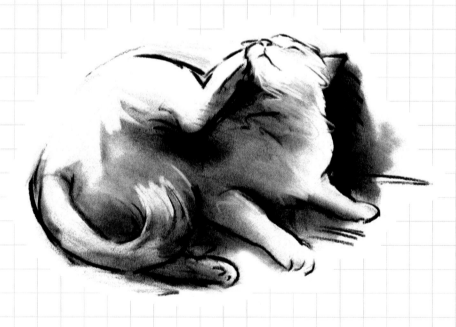

Microscopic organisms we cannot see are often more hazardous than dangers that can be seen by the human eye. Parasites can harm your cat's health and quality of life and sometimes even harm you and your family. Pesky parasites such as fleas can make life miserable for your pet and cause everyone in the home discomfort if the house becomes infested. Internal parasites such as heartworms and roundworms can cause health problems that will greatly diminish your cat's quality of life. The best measure of defense against parasites is to consult your veterinarian about preventive medications and ways to lessen the chance of parasites in your cat's environment. Pay close attention to strange behavior in your cat, which can often be a signal that a parasite is at work.

Q *How do I know if my cat has worms?*

A Cats get worms by eating raw meat, ingesting fleas, or from a queen, or mother cat, who passes worms through her placenta or milk to her kittens. If you notice your cat dragging, or scooting, her rear end along the floor, she could have any one of several varieties of worms. Tapeworm segments look like small pieces of rice when they pass in a cat's stool, but when they dry and stick to the hair under a cat's tail, they look like sesame seeds. Roundworms are longer, spaghetti-type worms that usually cause diarrhea, vomiting, or weight loss. Hookworms and whipworms are other long white worms that live in and damage the intestines. Regardless of the variety, worms are a nuisance and a threat to your cat's health. If live worms or segments are not observed externally, a microscopic fecal examination for worm eggs by your vet is the best way to discover if intestinal worms are present. No matter the circumstance, it is best to check with your veterinarian about diagnosis and treatment.

Once your vet identifies specific intestinal worms, he or she can administer oral or injectable medications to kill the parasites. Heavy worm loads in young animals can lead to dehydration and starvation, so animals with these clinical signs require additional supportive care. To help prevent intestinal worms in your cat, control fleas and make sure any meat fed to your cat is fully cooked.

Q *Can I get parasites from my cat?*

A Although unlikely, you can contract parasites such as roundworms, Toxoplasma gondii, and scabies from your cat if you don't practice good hygiene techniques. The best way to prevent exposing yourself to feline parasites is to wash your hands with soap and water after handling your cat, especially after cleaning the litter box. Since outdoor cats (whether it's your cat or someone else's) may eliminate in flowerbeds and yards, wear gloves when gardening to reduce your risk of contraction. Keep children's sand boxes covered when not in use so that cats do not use them as litter boxes. If your cat gets fleas, keep up with administering flea control medication. Fleas are considered a nuisance and will bite humans if they are hungry, but they cannot survive without a blood meal from a dog or cat.

Q *What other parasites can cause gastrointestinal disease?*

A Any cat experiencing vomiting and/or diarrhea should have a direct fecal smear examination in addition to a fecal float for parasites. Two protozoal parasites—coccidia and Giardia—can cause signs similar to those of intestinal worms. Protozoa are one-celled organisms, and certain species are capable of causing infections.

Coccidia infections occur when a cat ingests infected cysts from the environment or from raw meat. The cyst is one stage in an organism's life cycle. Infections in adult cats rarely cause any clinical signs or symptoms and resolve themselves without treatment. Kittens are more severely affected, and infections are associated with the stresses of weaning, living in a cattery or shelter, or shipping. Environmental contamination contributes to recurrent infection, so disinfecting as much of the home as possible, especially litter boxes with a dilute 1:32 bleach solution (1 part bleach to 32 parts water) is recommended. Affected cats respond to treatment with sulfa containing antibiotics and nutritional and fluid support in advanced cases.

Giardia infections behave similarly to coccidia infections with adult cats rarely affected and kittens developing significant clinical signs. Giardia is contracted from contaminated water or ingestion of infected cysts from the environment. Prevention involves environmental decontamination with dilute bleach and keeping the water supply clean. Metronidazole and fenbendazole are two of the most common drugs used in treatment of Giardia.

Q *What methods of flea control work best?*

A Fleas are parasites that must ingest a blood meal from a dog or cat to survive. They are a nuisance to your pet because they cause itchiness, carry tapeworms, and can cause anemia in heavy infestations.

The best flea control is achieved with products that are safe to humans and cats and have residual activity by continuing to kill fleas for a period of time after they have been applied. Flea control products available through your veterinarian, although expensive, are among the best. These include Bio-Spot, Program, Capstar, Advantage, Frontline, and Revolution. Your veterinarian can provide you with more information on the unique benefits of each and recommend a flea control program tailored to your cat's lifestyle and risk of exposure to fleas. Over-the-counter flea control products are also available, including topical treatments, shampoos, dips, sprays, mousses, and collars. Consult with your veterinarian to determine the best course of action for a flea infestation and/or prevention. Flea control products containing permethrins are toxic to cats and should never be used. Flea control products labeled for dogs should never be used on cats. If you choose to use over-the-counter products, read the labels carefully. There is one over-the-counter item every cat owner should own—a flea comb. This is a cheap and easy way to monitor your cat for fleas.

With the advent of effective products that kill adult fleas while they are on the cat, indoor flea control such as foggers, dehydrating powders, and house sprays are not often needed. The fleas die before they have the chance to reproduce and leave eggs in the environment.

Q *How do I know if my cat has mange?*

A Mange is a parasitic infection of the skin caused by mites. Mites are microscopic spiderlike parasites that cause itchiness and hair loss usually around the face and ears. Cats contract mange through exposure to other cats with the parasite. Indoor cats are not at risk for mange unless they are exposed to a new cat carrying mites. Keep an eye out for unfamiliar cats in your yard that may spread the infection.

The most common type of mange is Notoedres cati. This mite can create a self-limiting rash on a human but is otherwise specific to cats. Mange is cured through medical treatment with ivermectin, selamectin, or pyrethrins but can recur with repeated exposure. Treating your cat with the flea control product Revolution (selamectin) will also kill mange each month that it is used.

Q *Can I get ringworm from my cat?*

A Actually, ringworm is not a worm but a fungal infection. A few different types of fungi cause ringworm, but most often the cause of the infection is associated with the fungus Microsporum canis. Dermatophyte spores, ringworm causing fungi, are commonly found in dirt and can be tracked into indoor environments. Cats can carry the ringworm fungus without exhibiting the typical signs of dermatitis—scaling and crusting of the skin or nails and patches of hair loss. Be sure to consult your veterinarian if you suspect a ringworm problem. Increased risk for ringworm occurs in cats with weakened immune systems, those who live in crowded conditions such as shelters or catteries, and those who are stressed for any other reason since stress decreases the body's ability to fight infection. Young cats and breeds with long hair are more likely to be infected due to immature immune systems and genetics.

You can get ringworm through contact with your cat if she carries the fungus. Humans can also contract ringworm through infectious microscopic fungal spores that live in the environment.

Q If I'm pregnant, can I handle my cat?

A If you are planning a pregnancy, have yourself tested for the protozoal parasite toxoplasmosis first. If tests indicate previous exposure, there is no cause for concern. Toxoplasmosis is only a danger if an active infection occurs during pregnancy. If previously exposed, a woman will not develop a second infection. If you have not been exposed, doctors recommend that you avoid cleaning your cat's litter box so that you reduce the risk of exposure to Toxoplasma gondii. An infection with this parasite during pregnancy can lead to abortion, stillbirth, or birth of a sick child. Cats become infected with toxoplasmosis if they eat raw meat or prey carrying the parasite. They rarely develop any clinical signs but are responsible for spreading the organism through their feces. Women actually have a greater risk of exposure to toxoplasmosis if they handle raw meat or garden without wearing gloves and do not wash their hands thoroughly afterward because they could be exposed to infected cat feces in the dirt. During your pregnancy, have another family member clean the litter box, make sure you wash your hands after handling your cat, and do not allow your cat to walk on counters or surfaces where food is prepared.

Q What is cat scratch disease?

A Cat scratch disease is a bacterial infection caused by Bartonella henselae. Studies show that about 28 percent of cats in the United States test positive for the organism, although few become clinically ill. The ingestion of flea feces is more than likely the route of the cat's infection. Young cats (less than one year old), cats with fleas, and feral cats are more likely to be infected because they do not get flea control care. A bite or scratch from an infected cat can transmit the bacteria to humans. Clinical signs of infection for cats are similar to that of human signs of infection and include fever, lymph node enlargement, lethargy, and decreased appetite. Antibiotic treatment does not eliminate the infection from cats. Affected humans generally have a self-limiting disease that responds without treatment, but people with weakened immune systems need antibiotics and supportive care. To decrease your risk of exposure, control fleas on your cat, keep her toenails trimmed, and avoid rough play when scratching or biting can occur.

Q *Can my cat get Lyme disease?*

A Although cats living in areas where Lyme disease is found can test positive for the bacteria, they do not develop any apparent clinical signs. Cats cannot directly transmit the infection to humans. The spiral bacteria, Borrelia burgdorferi, causes Lyme disease. The deer tick Ixodes scapularis is the most common carrier of the disease. This tick transmits the bacteria by feeding (being attached to and sucking the blood of a person or another animal) for twenty-four to forty-eight hours. Humans and dogs are most likely to contract the disease, and cases predominantly occur in the northeastern United States. Signs of infection include fever, lameness, lymph node enlargement, loss of appetite, and malaise. To reduce your cat's exposure to Lyme disease, control tick infestation by keeping your cat indoors, checking outdoor cats daily for ticks and removing them, or using Frontline, which kills ticks.

Q *Is my cat at risk for heartworms?*

A Cats are at risk for developing heartworm disease if they live in areas where dogs are commonly infected. Mosquitoes carrying the parasite Dirofilaria immitis transmit heartworm disease. Therefore, outdoor cats, who have a higher exposure to mosquitoes, are most at risk. These cats should be placed on heartworm preventive medication as prescribed by your veterinarian.

Diagnosing heartworm disease is more difficult in cats than in dogs because fewer worms develop in infected cats, and many infected cats do not exhibit any clinical signs of infection. However, you might notice signs such as coughing, wheezing, lethargy, and vomiting in some infected cats. Your veterinarian can determine a clinical diagnosis through a combination of blood tests, X ray, and ultrasounds.

Treatment of heartworm disease focuses on relieving the clinical signs rather than eliminating the heartworms because cats cannot tolerate the same medications that kill adult worms in dogs. Adult heartworms live about two years, so if clinical signs are controlled and reinfection is prevented, the disease can be successfully treated. However, there is a chance that cats with heartworms can suddenly die from blood clots (arising from turbulent blood flow in the heart due to the presence of worms) lodging in the lungs.

Q *My cat has flea allergy dermatitis. What can I do to make my cat more comfortable?*

A Although fleas are itchy and annoying to a cat, some cats develop an allergic reaction to flea bites. For these cats, one flea bite is equal to a hundred bites in the discomfort and itchiness it creates. Cats with flea allergy dermatitis often have small scabs all over their skin, especially along their backs near their tail bases. They may lick and bite their own skin until it is bald and inflamed. Strict flea control is essential for preventing the initial reaction, and using the current, safe, spot-on products that kill adult fleas is recommended. Unfortunately, once the allergic reaction begins, medications are needed to calm the skin and treat any secondary infection. Veterinarians may use antihistamines, cortisone, and fatty acid supplements to treat inflammation and antibiotics for infections created when cats lick and scratch excessively.

Q *Why does my kitten still have loose stool after testing negative for parasites?*

A A single fecal check cannot rule out intestinal parasites. If the diarrhea continues, have the stool checked at least three times more with direct smears and flotations to test for parasites. It is a good idea regardless of the results to treat every kitten with a broad-spectrum deworming drug. Other options include feeding a bland diet to help firm the stool, then add other food into the diet.

Other causes of loose stool are dietary sensitivities, intestinal inflammation, and intestinal bacterial overgrowth. Some kittens develop intestinal bacterial overgrowth and respond to antibiotics and/or probiotics (supplements designed to reestablish normal intestinal bacterial flora). Long-term loose bowel movements are not normal for any cat, so be sure to consult your veterinarian.

Q *If my cat scratches her ears, does she have ear mites?*

A Ear mites are a problem in kittens and in adult cats who venture outdoors. Ear mites are microscopic bugs that live in ear canals and eat earwax and skin oils, which can cause itchiness, inflammation, and a buildup of waxy debris. Mites live for short periods of time off an animal in the ear environment, but are generally transmitted when one cat (or dog) with ear mites comes in physical contact (crawling, falling over, rubbing) with another cat. Your veterinarian can easily identify mites either by otoscopic examination of the ears or by microscopic examination of ear swabs. These tests verify the presence of live mites and/or eggs.

If ear mites are definitively diagnosed, they can be eliminated as long as there is no additional exposure to the bugs; therefore, all dogs and cats in the household need to be treated at the same time. There are many effective treatments for mites, including medicated eardrops, internal treatment with ivermectin, and topical treatment with selamectin (Revolution). Recurrent ear problems in indoor cats are more likely due to yeast infections or allergies—problems arising from environmental conditions and individual sensitivities. Ear mites are not transmissible to humans.

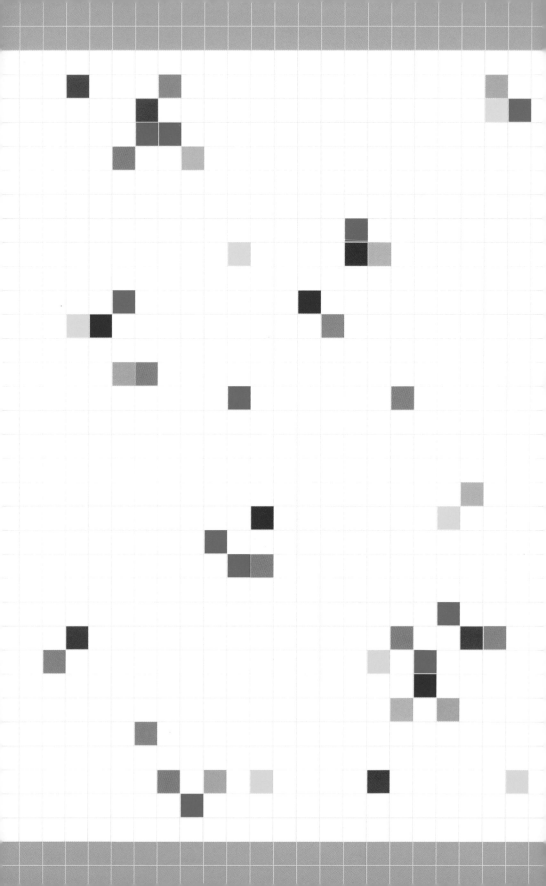

CHAPTER 4

Vaccines and Routine Care

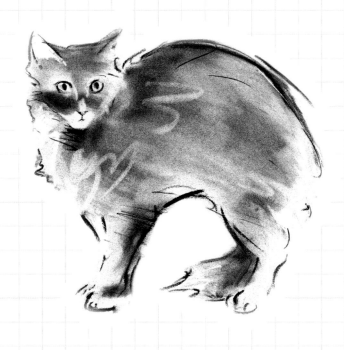

Part of your responsibility as a cat owner is to make sure your pet is up to date on all necessary vaccinations and that annual examinations, medications, and routine care are maintained. Like a small child, a new kitten will need a battery of vaccines at the beginning of his life and follow-up care throughout his life. Medications may, at some point, also play a part in your cat's health care, and administering medications can sometimes be a challenge to a cat owner. Observe changes in your cat's health and communicate with your veterinarian. The two of you can work together to ensure that your cat enjoys a good quality of life.

Q *How do I administer medicine to my cat?*

A A positive attitude and a few techniques are all you need to medicate your cat successfully. Before you administer a medication to your cat, make sure that your veterinarian explains the dosing directions clearly so that you understand what you need to do.

Almost every medication comes in tablet or capsule form, so if you can master pilling, you are in good shape for administering other types of medications. I recommend placing your cat on a counter or table when administering medication. This puts the cat at a level that is more comfortable for you to handle, and it takes away the cat's ability to squirm and run away. Hold your cat's upper cheekbones with your thumb and index finger and then point your cat's nose toward the ceiling—this automatically causes your cat to open his mouth. With your free hand, pop the pill over his tongue, then use a syringe without a needle to squirt water into his mouth. Recent veterinary studies show that pills stay lodged in the cat's esophagus for extended periods of time if they are not followed with a small swallow of water.

Because many drugs are bitter or start dissolving in the cat's mouth, you may have a hard time with pilling, but there are numerous tricks that can make pilling easier for you and your cat. Pills can be coated with butter or margarine to disguise taste. Cats who like hairball lubricant can usually be tricked into swallowing a pill that is coated with it. Bitter pills are easily administered when placed in gel caps. Pill guns (plastic pill administering devices) are useful to push the pill over the back of the tongue if you are unsuccessful with your fingers or your cat attempts to bite. Foaming and gagging after oral medications is common in cats, especially if the event is stressful or the cat doesn't like the taste of the medication. Occasionally, owners try to administer a pill by crushing or mixing the pill into canned food, or they try making a small "meatball" of canned food with a pill in the center, but the cat's keen sense of smell and taste usually alerts him to a foreign substance in the food, and he will avoid eating it.

Liquid medications are easier for most owners to administer. You don't need to pry open a cat's mouth to administer liquids, but simply place the tip of the dropper or syringe in the corner of the cat's mouth, tilt his head up slightly, and squirt slowly. Some liquid medications require refrigeration, and they taste better to cats when cold.

Many cats are extremely difficult to medicate, and unfortunately many of the drugs utilized in veterinary medicine are human drugs, which are not manufactured in feline-friendly forms. Because of this, veterinarians are increasingly utilizing compounding pharmacies, which reformulate drugs into gel caps, chewable treats, flavored liquids, and even transdermal gels. If you are unable to medicate your cat using standard techniques, ask your veterinarian about compounded medications.

Q *Should I vaccinate my cat? If so, how often?*

A Having your cat vaccinated annually used to be standard veterinary practice. The veterinary profession, however, has begun to question the need for annual vaccinations. This is in light of new information regarding the duration of immunity from disease and the adverse vaccine reactions such as tumors that may be associated with vaccination.

The American Association of Feline Practitioners created its first vaccine guidelines in 1998. The general recommendations assess an individual cat's risk of infection as the cornerstone to developing that animal's vaccine protocol. The three items the owner and veterinarian need to evaluate are the cat, the cat's environment, and the infectious agents to which the cat may be exposed.

The guidelines also distinguish core and noncore vaccines. A core vaccine is recommended for all cats. There are two core vaccines for cats and it's recommended that all cats get these vaccines. One protects against the feline rhinotracheitis, calici, and panleukopenia viruses and is referred to as FRCP, the other protects against rabies. The general recommendation is to administer the FRCP vaccine to kittens six to eight weeks of age, then every three to four weeks until they are twelve weeks old. A booster should follow one year later, then every three years. The rabies vaccine can be administered to kittens at least twelve weeks old, again one year later, and then every three years. Exceptions exist regarding this protocol, which includes state laws that dictate the requirements for rabies vaccination. A noncore vaccine, such as feline leukemia virus (FeLV), may be appropriate in certain situations, but is not recommended for all cats.

The guidelines address recommended sites of vaccination as well for each of the common vaccines. Different vaccines may best be administered at different sites. Standardized vaccine sites help identify causes and aid in the treatment of adverse reactions. The recommended sites for administering vaccines are: FRCP vaccines over the right shoulder, rabies in the right rear leg, and FeLV vaccines (if needed) in the left rear leg; all administered as far away from the trunk as practical. Vaccinating between the shoulder blades is not recommended because if a tumor arises in this location, it is almost impossible to remove.

Q What is the FRCP vaccine?

A The letters stand for feline rhinotracheitis, calici, and panleukopenia. This is the cat vaccine that all cats should receive as kittens, and then on a schedule as adults. It is also called the three-way vaccine because it protects against three diseases.

Feline panleukopenia is a virus that is usually fatal to infected cats. It is shed in feces, transmitted through fecal-oral contact, and spreads through poor hygiene. It can contaminate cages, eating bowls, and litter boxes. Most vaccines containing this virus stimulate complete protective immunity. Clinical signs associated with panleukopenia include fever, anorexia, vomiting, or diarrhea. The most characteristic laboratory finding is an extremely low white blood cell count. Death can be rapid due to severe dehydration and electrolyte imbalances.

Feline herpesvirus (feline rhinotracheitis) and feline calicivirus are estimated to cause up to 90 percent of upper respiratory disease cases in cats. These diseases are rarely fatal but are extremely prevalent. Transmission occurs through sneezing and aerosol spread of droplets, by direct contact, and by contaminated objects. Common signs of these diseases include sneezing, anorexia, and conjunctivitis (inflammation of the mucosal tissue around the eye). Cats can develop chronic herpesvirus infections that cause long-term, intermittent bouts of sneezing and conjunctivitis. Feline calicivirus infection can also cause limping or severe gum disease. Vaccination against these viruses does not prevent infection, but it does reduce the severity of the associated clinical symptoms. In addition to the traditional form of vaccination (an injection), a topical vaccination is available for these viruses. Topical vaccines may be administered in an intranasal (in the nose) or intraocular (in the eye) manner.

Q *What are feline leukemia and feline AIDS?*

A Feline leukemia virus (FeLV) is a potentially fatal virus to cats. It is passed by direct cat-to-cat contact and by a queen to her kittens. Clinical signs associated with FeLV are nonspecific and can range from anemia to immunosuppression to tumor formation. FeLV can cause latent infections that may not produce clinical signs for months or years. Testing and identifying FeLV positive cats is essential to controlling the infection. Cats at risk for exposure to FeLV include outdoor cats; stray cats; feral cats; multicat households where newcomers are brought in without iso-

43

lation and testing; FeLV positive households; and households with unknown FeLV status. Vaccination is recommended for cats who test negative but who live in environments where these possibilities for exposure exist. Some veterinarians recommend that all kittens receive an initial FeLV vaccination series since their risk exposure may not yet be defined (i.e. may or may not go outside in the future). Initial vaccination for this noncore vaccine is at least eight weeks of age, then four weeks later, and then annually. Changes in your cat's home environment could increase or decrease his risk; subsequent vaccination decisions should be based on these risks. Vaccination ensures fair to good immunity.

Feline AIDS is caused by the feline immunodeficiency virus (FIV), which is strictly a feline virus but similar to human immunodeficiency virus (HIV). The virus suppresses the immune system, but infected cats don't deteriorate as rapidly as cats infected with FeLV; many infected cats live normal life spans. The virus is usually passed through cat bites, so outside cats who fight are most at risk for infection. A vaccine for FIV was developed in 2002, but it does not protect against all strains of the virus. Healthy cats vaccinated against FIV test positive when given routine viral screening tests, so the results can be dangerously misinterpreted. At this time, vaccination is only recommended in situations deemed necessary by your veterinarian.

Good diagnostic tests exist that screen for these viruses; therefore, you should know the FeLV and FIV status of your cat so that you know if your cat is potentially contagious or may get sick and die.

Q *How can my cat contract rabies?*

A Rabies is a virus contracted through contact with infected saliva, usually through bite wounds or mucous membranes (eyes and mouth). Cats most often contract the infection after being bitten by infected raccoons, skunks, foxes, or bats.

The incubation period of a rabies infection is two to six weeks. This is the time between exposure and development of clinical signs.

During the first two to four days of signs, cats act aggressively and unpredictably and pose a high risk for human exposure. Rabies is a core vaccine (recommended for all cats) because of the potential for a rabid cat bite to a human and because the infection is fatal for the infected animal. Each state has different laws regulating rabies vaccination that should be upheld.

Q *How will I know if my cat is having a reaction to a vaccine?*

A Common reactions to vaccines are a low-grade fever, decreased appetite, and lethargy, all which usually resolve within twenty-four hours. Some cats vomit. The signs of a more serious reaction needing immediate veterinary care are fainting and difficulty breathing. Vaccine reactions are treated with antihistamines, cortisone, and other supportive care.

Monitor your cat if he develops lumps where the vaccine was injected. Normally, a lump will resolve itself within four weeks of vaccination. If it does not, a biopsy may be necessary. An increasing incidence of a type of tumor called fibrosarcoma has been noted in locations where vaccines are routinely administered to cats. Research is being conducted and a national veterinary task force exists to determine what the relationship is between vaccines and sarcomas. The incidence of vaccine site sarcomas is estimated at 1-3 out of every 10,000 vaccines administered, an extremely low number. The veterinary community feels that the risk of disease from not vaccinating is much higher than the risks associated with vaccinating, but a rethinking of how, when, where, and why we vaccinate cats has resulted. Ask your veterinarian about the details on fibrosarcoma before you decide not to vaccinate your cat. Chances are, she will advise you that the benefits of vaccinations outweigh the risks.

Once a cat has a vaccine reaction, you should take precautions to prevent future problems. You can premedicate the cat with an antihistamine fifteen minutes before the vaccination, split up multiple vaccines by giving only one per month, and discontinue future vaccination.

45

Q *What other vaccines are there?*

A There are some vaccinations that may not be necessary for your cat unless he is in a high-risk situation. The vaccination guidelines created by the American Association of Feline Practitioners considers the following vaccines to be non-core and are recommended based on a cat's specific risk level:

• **Chlamydia**, a bacterial infection that causes upper respiratory disease, chlamydia is the last component in the FRCPC, or four-way vaccine. Transmission occurs through direct cat-to-cat contact. The most common clinical symptom is severe conjunctivitis. Vaccination does not prevent infection, but it can lessen the clinical symptoms. The prevalence of Chlamydophila psittaci in the United States is considered to be low. At this time, the duration of immunity from the vaccination is unknown, but annual vaccination is recommended for cats at risk.

• **Feline Infectious Peritonitis (FIP)** is another potentially fatal virus to cats. This virus' mode of transmission is not definitively known, but the current theory is that it develops in certain cats who have oral or nasal contact with feces infected with feline enteric corona virus (FECV). A queen may transmit the disease to her kittens as well. FECV is not a life threatening virus, but it is highly contagious to cats. Diarrhea is a common symptom of infection. In certain cats, FECV may mutate and become FIP, but it depends on circumstances, including age (a one-year-old being most susceptible because of a less mature immune system), breed, genetics, general health, immune status, and environmental stresses. Reliable screening tests for FIP do not exist; therefore, assessing the vaccine's effectiveness is difficult. The cases of FIP in pet households are low, but cats are at risk if they live in households where FIP has been previously diagnosed. Initially, this noncore vaccine can be administered in two doses, three to four weeks apart for cats over sixteen weeks, then annually.

• *Microsporum canis* is a fungus that causes ringworm. M. canis can affect cats and humans, but generally infections are limited to skin rashes. Complete treatment aimed at preventing and eliminating the fungus involves oral, topical, and home environment treatment. The vaccine can be used in a complete control program but is not recommended for every cat.

• *Bordetella bronchiseptica* is the bacteria that causes kennel cough in dogs and has been shown to cause upper respiratory disease and pneumonia in cats. The vaccine is not recommended for routine use, but may be considered for cats who enter or live in households where the organism has caused clinical disease.

• *Giardia Lamblia* is a protozoal parasite that causes diarrhea. This vaccine is not recommended for routine use, but may be considered as part of a treatment program in multiple cat environments with clinical infections of Giardia.

• A vaccine for FIV was approved by the USDA in March 2002. Studies show that about two-thirds of the cats who were vaccinated were protected against two out of four strains of the virus, whereas three-quarters of unvaccinated cats became infected. One potential problem with this vaccine is that current diagnostic tests cannot distinguish vaccinated from infected cats; they can only be differentiated with virus isolation, a complicated test not widely available or standardized. At this time, routine use of the vaccine is not recommended.

Q *When will my kitten lose his baby teeth?*

A Cats, like humans, develop two sets of teeth. Kittens develop their twenty-six baby teeth deciduous from four to six weeks of age, at which time they are also weaned from nursing and begin to eat solid food. Your cat will start to lose his baby teeth and develop his thirty adult teeth from four to seven months of age. Teething kittens are more "oral" and tend to bite and chew on everything—including their owner's hands and feet, so be on the lookout for excessive biting. Most owners do not notice when their cats lose their teeth because the teeth are usually swallowed and passed in the stool.

Q *What happens when a cat is declawed?*

A Declawing is a major surgery and not just a removal or cutting back of the toenails. Declawing is the surgical amputation of the last joint in each toe of a cat's foot. The entire third phalanx bone of each toe must be removed to prevent nail formation. It is an irreversible procedure that is more painful for heavier and mature cats.

Some veterinarians perform an alternative surgical procedure called a digital tenotomy. Although considered less painful to the cat since bone is not removed, it requires more owner maintenance. In this procedure, the tendons that control retraction of each nail are cut so that the cat loses her ability to claw. The nails are left dangling in place so they do not wear down as they would if the cat could still claw, and length cannot be controlled without frequent trimming.

In both cases, there is nothing an owner can do to ease the cat's pain other than administer pain medication prescribed by the veterinarian. Alternatives to declawing include properly training your cat to use a scratching post, trimming your cat's nails every couple of weeks, and applying protective vinyl nail caps.

Q *What form of identification will help my cat get found if he gets lost?*

A Whether your cat goes outside or stays inside, identification is a good idea in case of an emergency. Most cats tolerate wearing a collar with an identification tag or plate, especially if trained at a young age. However, collars pose a risk for active cats. If the collar gets caught, the cat can be harmed, so a breakaway style collar is best.

Another option for identification is a microchip, which a veterinarian injects under the skin to provide permanent identification. Each chip carries a unique number that can be traced to a specific cat. The downside of a microchip is that it can be read only with a special scanner. Anyone who finds your cat will not be able to tell who the cat belongs to unless he or she takes him to the vet to be scanned and identified. Tattoos and eartags are other less commonly used modes of identification available.

Q *Can routine vaccines cause cancer?*

A Vaccine-associated feline sarcomas are malignant tumors that occur rarely in some cats. At this time there is no way to predict the occurrence because the specific cause remains uncertain, but there are some things you can do to reduce the risk for your cat.

Ask your veterinarian to use single-agent vaccines when possible. This will allow your veterinarian to develop a vaccine plan specific for your cat and stagger vaccination visits. You can also work with your veterinarian to make sure she gives each different vaccine in the American Association of Feline Practitioner's recommended location on your cat's body. That way, the vet can track any problems and associate them with the corresponding vaccination location.

When you and your cat are home, examine him for any knots on or around the vaccination site. Small bumps are normal immediately after vaccination, but should not be present weeks after he has received his shots.

Though there is a small risk for vaccine-associated feline sarcoma, keep in mind that the benefits of vaccinating your cat far outweigh the risks. You play a vital role in keeping your cat healthy and disease-free, and vaccination is a key element in his overall health.

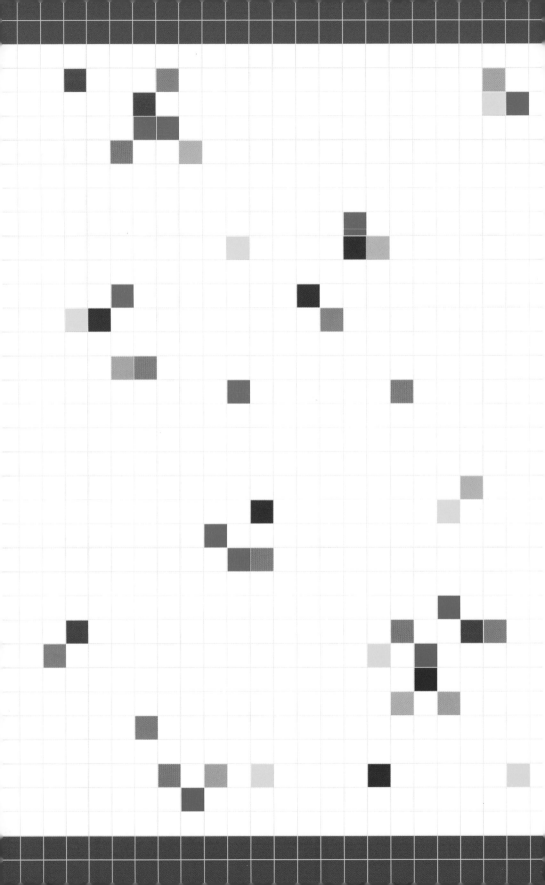

CHAPTER 5

First Aid and Emergency Care

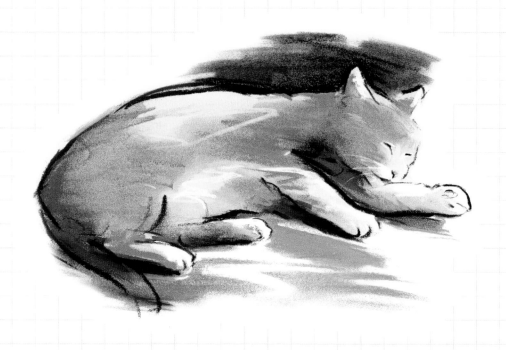

Not everything can be cured with a home remedy or ignored until the next morning. Sometimes cats need immediate emergency medical attention. Often this means that you will have to take your cat to an emergency clinic and work with an unfamiliar vet or technician. Rest assured that this is far preferable to waiting until the next day so you can see your regular vet—your cat's well-being should be the top priority. To prevent emergencies, stay vigilant about your cat's whereabouts and simply use good judgment. For example, if you live in a hot, humid climate, it's a good idea to always keep your cat well hydrated and have a cooling plan in place if she gets overheated. If your cat makes the neighborhood rounds each evening, check her body for signs of a cat fight when she returns home. Your awareness is your cat's strongest ally since she can't verbalize her pain.

Q *How do I find an emergency animal clinic?*

A You may be faced with an emergency situation with your cat at times when your regular veterinary hospital is closed. There are various options for emergency care. Plan ahead by asking your veterinarian what options he or she has available or recommends and keep this information handy for future use. Veterinary emergency services are listed in your yellow pages. In most emergencies you may need to go to the closest facility. Ideally you will want to find a full service emergency clinic that has a veterinarian and technician on duty and ready to handle any emergency. Most emergency clinics are not linked to regular daytime veterinary practices and are open after hours and on weekends and holidays. Emergency services are more expensive than routine care, so be sure that you understand the recommended charges and treatments so that you can make a good decision for your cat's care.

Q *How can I tell if my cat has a fever?*

A Cats with fevers are generally lethargic and have no appetite. Although popular culture has led us to believe that a healthy cat has a cold, wet nose and therefore a warm, dry nose is indicative of a fever, this is not always true. Many conditions including environmental temperature and the cat's state of hydration affect how cold and wet a nose is. If your cat's ears feel hot to the touch she may have a fever. The only reliable way to determine if your cat has a fever is by taking her temperature. A cat's normal body temperature is typically between 100.5° F and 102.5° F. Human ear thermometers are not reliable for taking your cat's temperature due to the way they are calibrated and the different shape of a cat's ear canal. There are special ear thermometers for animals that are useful with cats, but they cost several hundred dollars. The best and most economical way for you to take your cat's temperature is by using a pediatric rectal glass or digital thermometer. Taking your cat's temperature usually takes two people: one to restrain the cat and the other to insert the thermometer.

Conventional thermometers should be lubricated with petroleum jelly or water soluble lubricants such as K-Y Jelly and left in the rectum for two minutes. Digital thermometers are lubricated and left in the rectum until they beep. On hot days or if a cat is stressed, her body temperature may reach 103.5° F. Veterinarians are concerned when temperatures reach 104° F or higher. Aspirin is not routinely used to bring down a fever in a cat. If your cat does have a fever you should bring her to your veterinarian as soon as possible.

 Q *Is it safe to give my cat aspirin?*

A You should never administer aspirin to a cat without a veterinarian's approval. Cats do not metabolize aspirin, acetaminophen, ibuprofen, or other nonsteroidal anti-inflammatory drugs (NSAIDs) well, and giving your cat one of these substances can cause toxicities or even death. Regular aspirin is 325 mg, and healthy cats only tolerate low dose aspirin or children's aspirin (81-83 mg) once every three days. If your cat must take aspirin you and your vet need to discuss a treatment plan.

Aspirin is most commonly used in cats for pain relief after trauma, chronic conditions such as arthritis, and to prevent blood clots. Aspirin should be given with food to decrease stomach irritation as some cats experience side effects, including vomiting, loss of appetite, or even bruising. Cats who ingest higher doses of aspirin may become depressed, anorexic, anemic, vomit, or develop stomach bleeding or bone marrow suppression. Intensive veterinary care should be administered if your cat accidentally ingests aspirin or any other NSAID.

Q *What should I do if my cat gets into a fight?*

A If you observe your cat in a fight, try to break it up by making loud noises, squirting the cats with a hose, or intervening with a broom. Owners using their hands and feet to try to separate fighting cats can be bitten severely. After the fight, examine your cat's body and try to evaluate whether any punctures or lacerations are present. Finding punctures is difficult, especially on long-haired cats. Clumped tufts of hair or moist areas are indicators of wounds. Clean any puncture wound with hydrogen peroxide. A veterinarian should suture any sizeable lacerations.

If you discover wounds and swelling a few days after a fight, take your cat to a veterinarian. Infected wounds that fester for a few days often develop into abscesses. Once an abscess develops, antibiotics alone cannot cure the infection. Abscesses require sedation or anesthesia, lancing, surgical closure, and antibiotic treatment. If there is a large pocket of infection, the veterinarian will place a drain in the infected area for a few days after the surgery and put an Elizabethan collar on the cat to prevent her from pulling out the drain or licking the surgery site. An Elizabeth collar is a large lampshade shaped plastic disk that prevents animals from licking, chewing, or biting their bodies. The cat can still perform normal daily tasks, like eating from a dish.

Outdoor cats should be vaccinated against FeLV and rabies, as well as FIV if recommended by your veterinarian since these viruses can be passed during a cat fight. Frequent fighters should be tested annually for FeLV and FIV. Territoriality and sexual behaviors trigger cat fights, so neuter your outdoor cat as soon as possible.

Q *What should I do if I cut a toenail too short and it bleeds?*

A If you regularly trim your cat's toenails, it is a good idea to have some cautery powder or styptic pencils available. These items will stop bleeding. If you don't have either of these items available, touch the bleeding nail to an ice cube. This will cause the blood vessel to constrict and bleeding to slow. Cats lose a lot of blood from toenails that are broken or cut too short, but a cat will not lose so much blood that it's dangerous.

When trimming your cat's nails, use nail clippers specifically designed for pets. Cat nails are round, so when human nail clippers are used a cat's nail gets crushed. If you look for the quick (the blood vessel in the nail that looks like a pink triangle) before cutting and cut below it, you will not have a problem with bleeding. If you have a problem seeing your cat's toenails, vertically press the pad of each toe between your thumb and forefinger: this will exteriorize the nail. Always trim the nails in the same sequence so that you don't miss any of them. Cats normally have five toes on each front foot and four on each back. To play it safe when starting out, only cut the tip of the nail, and when you're more confident cut more. Toenails grow back every two to three weeks.

Q *What should I do if my cat gets overheated?*

A Overheating is a dangerous condition that arises when a cat is trapped in a car or room without ventilation, when a sick cat lies too long in the sun, or when a cat gets dried with a hair dryer on high heat. Overheated cats can have a body temperature of over 106° F (normal temperature is 100.5° F–102.5° F); temperatures this high lead to internal organ damage. Overheated cats pant, drool, and can be so weak that they faint.

If you think your cat is overheated and you notice the above signs, it is important bring down your cat's body temperature quickly and safely. To do so, place the cat in a sink or tub filled with cold water or spray your cat down with cold water. Another alternative is to soak the paws and armpits in rubbing alcohol. This wets the fur and causes evaporation. Take your cat's temperature every fifteen minutes because your cat's temperature can drop too low very quickly. Transport the cat to a veterinarian as soon as you can—dripping wet if possible. Your veterinarian needs to examine your cat for signs of shock and administer treatment, if needed.

Q *What should I do if I suspect my cat has fractured a limb?*

A If you suspect that your cat has fractured a limb, use extreme care when picking her up or checking her because she may bite you. A broken bone is a painful injury. If you see your cat hopping around on three legs, it is a good indication a limb is broken since cats do not put any weight on a broken limb. Swelling can be a sign of a fracture, but it is also indicative of a bite wound or insect sting. A fracture where part of the bone is exposed is called a compound, or open fracture, which you should cover with a clean towel for protection. If you suspect any type of fracture, take your cat to a veterinarian as soon as possible.

Regardless of where a fracture is located, X rays are needed to determine the severity of the break and the number of bone fragments that are present. These factors are crucial in determining which options are available in caring for the break. Depending on the location, bones that are cracked but not displaced can be splinted. More serious fractures require pinning, bone plating, or external fixation. In circumstances where bones are crushed or economics prevent proper treatment, your vet may recommend limb amputation.

Q *How dangerous is antifreeze to cats?*

A Antifreeze is one of the most toxic chemicals owners have in their homes. Ingestion, even just a small amount, is lethal. The active chemical in antifreeze, ethylene glycol, destroys a cat's kidneys. It is so toxic, that unless exposure is recognized and treated within three to four hours of ingestion, it is unlikely that the cat's life can be saved. Clinical signs of toxicity are depression, vomiting, anorexia, hypothermia, stumbling, muscle tremors, or seizures.

If you suspect your cat has ingested antifreeze, take her to the vet immediately. The vet will do a routine blood panel. Although this will not specifically diagnose ethylene glycol poisoning, it will indicate that problems with the kidneys and liver exist. If ingestion is suspected, a special blood test is available for the chemical, and urinalysis usually reveals calcium oxalate crystals that are diagnostic for ethylene glycol ingestion. Once the cause is determined, treatment focuses on combating shock and maintaining kidney function. An antidote to ethylene glycol is intravenous ethanol, but if this is not administered quickly after ingestion it is not helpful. To prevent antifreeze exposure, fix any leaking car radiators and thoroughly clean up any antifreeze spills. Antifreeze containing propylene glycol is a safe alternative that won't harm your cat.

Q *What should I do if my cat eats something that's bad for her?*

A You should consult your veterinarian or the Animal Poison Control Center at 888-426-4435 if you suspect your cat has eaten something harmful. As finicky as cats are, they sometimes ingest items that are toxic or unable to pass through their gastrointestinal tracts. Some cats will eat objects such as plastic, buttons, coins, rubber stoppers, or ribbons. A cat who eats any one of these objects may vomit or the object will either pass or cause an obstruction depending on it's size and shape. Lengths of ribbons, thread, dental floss, and yarn are dangerous if a cat ingests a piece longer than a couple of inches. These items are called linear foreign bodies and they cause the intestine to become accordion-pleated with compromised blood flow.

Items such as bones, metal, and most rubber or hard plastic objects show up well on X rays. It is more difficult to see other types of objects that can be less clearly defined. Ultrasound can aid diagnosis, but on its own it is not solely reliable for diagnosis of a foreign body. A barium upper GI series, also can show an obstruction.

Q *What should I do if a bee or wasp stings my cat?*

A If you know that your cat was stung, try to examine the area and remove the stinger if it is still present. Antihistamines reduce swelling if given within an hour of the sting—the sooner the better. Owners can give half of a 25 mg diphenhydramine (Benadryl) or half of a 4 mg chlorpheniramine (Chlortrimetron) orally to an adult cat. Your veterinarian will likely prescribe a combination of cortisone and antihistamine to stop the swelling and reaction. The swelling usually lasts a few days after a sting.

Most cats stung by bees or wasps develop only local swelling and irritation but do not develop anaphylaxis (allergic shock reaction). Signs of anaphylaxis from a sting are difficulty breathing, vomiting, drooling, and weakness. If any of these signs are evident, seek immediate veterinary care.

Q *What should I do if my cat is hit by a car?*

A Do not wait to take your cat to the veterinarian if you suspect she has been hit by a car. Sometimes a cat can walk away from a car accident, and this can be extremely dangerous because she may not display outward signs of injury. Cats can sustain severe internal injuries and look unharmed on the outside.

If your cat is hit by a car, call your veterinarian immediately or an emergency animal hospital if it is after regular business hours. Make sure your cat is breathing and check for a heartbeat. Check her body for any external wounds and stop the bleeding by applying pressure with gauze pads or a clean towel. If you suspect your cat has sustained a broken bone, try to limit your contact with the limb so you do not create a more serious injury. Carefully place your cat into a large enough box to lay her flat and get her to the veterinarian as quickly and safely as possible.

Q *What does it mean if there is blood in my cat's stool?*

A Although it is alarming to see blood in a cat's stool, it actually occurs fairly frequently. Possible causes include parasites, constipation, colitis, dietary indiscretion or anal gland infection. It is extremely unlikely that blood in your cat's stool is a sign of life-threatening disease.

Adding fiber to a a cat's diet with a psyllium-containing supplement or administering a lubricating hairball remedy are two possible treatments if no medical problems are found. If episodes of blood in the stool becomre more frequent, other tests such as a lower GI endoscopy might be needed. Black stools indicate bleeding in the stomach or in the first part of the intestine, and this is usually a more serious condition that warrants immediate medical attention.

Q *My cat is rapidly losing weight. What can this mean?*

A Rapid weight loss in a cat may be due to kidney disease. Loss of kidney function is common in cats 10 years and older. Chronic tubulointerstitial nephritis is the medical term for the typical progressive degeneration of the kidneys. Owners might suspect kidney disease if they notice increased thirst, increased urination, and weight loss in their pet. To test for kidney disease, blood and urine tests are performed by your veterinarian. These tests do not begin to show abnormal results until about two-thirds of the kidney function has been compromised.

Most cats with chronic kidney disease, also called chronic renal insufficiency, will respond for a period of time to fluid supplementation, control of electrolytes (minerals in the blood), and diet. Unfortunately, this disease cannot be cured. The earlier kidney disease is diagnosed, the greater the possibility of successful long term management. Owners are frequently trained by their veterinarian to give their cat injections of sterile fluids under the skin in order to maintain fluid balance and keep the cat feeling good. How quickly kidney disease progresses is variable, but regular monitoring by your veterinarian will determine the prognosis.

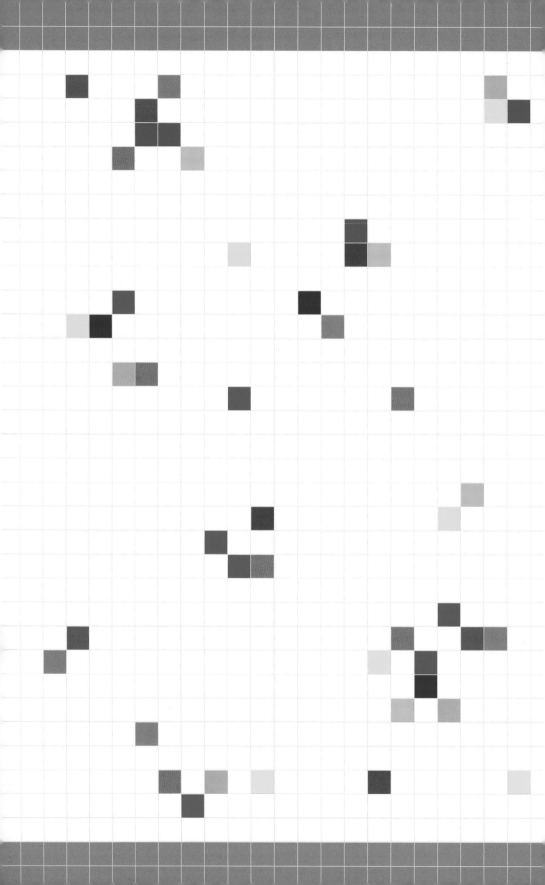

CHAPTER 6

Reproduction

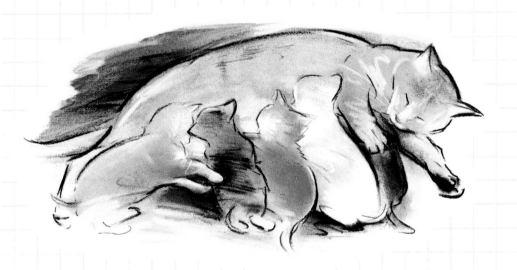

Pet overpopulation is an enormous problem that is compounded every time a cat owner makes the choice not to sterilize his or her pet. Many pet owners think if they have a house cat, there is no issue with unwanted reproduction, which may not always be the case. Sterilization makes cats better pets because it helps prevent unwanted behaviors and eliminates certain health risks. Anything can happen, so the best bet is to be prepared and do your part to control the cat population. If you do wish for your cat to reproduce, consult with your veterinarian about the safest methods.

Q *At what age can I sterilize my pet?*

A Many veterinarians routinely sterilize cats at about six months of age, but more experienced veterinarians are able to perform surgery at an earlier age (eight to twenty weeks old). The spay surgery for a female cat is called an ovariohysterectomy. This procedure removes the uterus and both ovaries. The neuter surgery for a male cat is called a castration; both testicles are surgically removed. You can use the information below as a guide, but you should discuss the best time to sterilize your cat with your veterinarian.

Ideally you want to sterilize your cat before he or she reaches puberty. Most cats reach puberty around six to seven months of age, but during the spring mating season, some cats mature more quickly. The typical signs of sexual maturity in a female cat are restlessness, rolling on the ground, and increased crying or other vocalizations. Some owners think that their female cats roll around and act as if they are in pain, but hormones are triggering this behavior, which is painless. Female cats are seasonally polyestrous, meaning they go through multiple heat cycles during the year—mostly between February and October. Unless a cat becomes pregnant or is otherwise stimulated to ovulate, she can cycle every two to three weeks, which becomes annoying to owners. Signs of maturity in male cats are agitation, increased territoriality, attempts to dart outside (and look for a girlfriend), an increase in the size of the cheeks and lower jaw, and a foul, musky urine odor.

Some owners worry that sterilizing will make their cats fat and lazy, but cats become fat and lazy due to overfeeding and lack of exercise. When you sterilize your cat, you need to adjust the amount of food you feed him or her as sterilized cats have a slower metabolic rate. If your cat continues to gain weight, consult your veterinarian about a healthy weight loss plan.

Early age sterilization is becoming more common, especially with breeders and shelters to help combat pet overpopulation. By sterilizing early there is little chance a cat will get pregnant or impregnate other cats, and it eliminates the need for you to remember when your cat is close to puberty and has to be spayed or neutered. Studies show that cats who undergo early sterilization are as healthy and have the same longevity as cats who are sterilized at a later age. Extra precautions need to be taken with younger cats since their immune systems are not as strong: anesthesia doses need adjusting and the body temperature needs more regulation during and after surgery because hypothermia due to a lack of body fat is more likely.

Q *Should I let my female cat go through a heat cycle before I spay her?*

A It is actually healthier for a cat to be sterilized before heat cycles begin. Cats that start going through heat are at a much higher risk of developing mammary cancer later in life. Cats that are sterilized before cycling have virtually no risk of the disease. Going through a heat cycle does not improve a cat's personality, and sterilizing does not take away any desirable aspects of a cat's personality. Some owners worry that sterilizing will make their cat fat and lazy, but cats become fat and lazy due to overfeeding. Sterilized cats have a slower metabolic rate, so feeding needs adjustment.

Since they have no uterus, spayed female cats have no risk of metritis or pyometra. Metritis is a treatable uterine infection. Pyometra is a potentially life threatening infection of the uterus that can occur in intact females, especially if they are not bred.

Q *Why should I neuter my male cat?*

A There are many good reasons for neutering male cats. The first good reason is that intact male cats contribute to pet overpopulation and millions of cats are destroyed every year because they have no homes. Even if you want to keep an intact male inside, chances are he will get out at some point because his hormones tell him to search for a mate.

The second reason for neutering male cats is that they make much better pets. Neutering does not alter the good parts of a male cat's personality, but it does decrease aggressive and territorial tendencies. Intact male cats are more likely to get into cat fights, which increases their risk of exposure to disease and increases the owners cost of keeping them healthy.

The third reason to neuter a cat is that intact males are more likely to spray, which is an undesirable behavior for an indoor cat. Once a cat starts spraying, neutering will help, but there is no guarantee it will eliminate the problem. A young male cat's urine odor is not very strong, but after puberty, it changes to a foul smell that ruins anything it comes in contact with. Deodorizers and neutralizers help, but they cannot eliminate the smell of tomcat urine.

Q *How long is a cat pregnant?*

A The gestation period is the time that a cat is pregnant, which runs sixty-three to sixty-nine days. Owners do not realize that a cat is pregnant until she is about halfway through the pregnancy. Pregnant cats stop their heat cycles and their nipples "pink up" about two weeks into the pregnancy. The body temperature of a queen, an intact female, drops to 99°F about twenty-four hours before she has kittens. If you suspect your cat is pregnant, track her temperature rectally twice daily.

An abdominal palpation can confirm that your cat is pregnant if she is three to four weeks along; an ultrasound can diagnose pregnancy earlier. At about day fifty-four of the pregnancy, X rays can determine the number of fetuses present. X rays are not harmful to the fetuses or the queen. If a first time queen has not gone into labor by the sixty-seventh day of gestation, a veterinarian should examine her.

Q *Can my cat get pregnant while she is nursing a litter?*

A Unfortunately, the answer is yes. Once your cat has given birth, she begins her estrus (heat) cycles again. Therefore, if your cat is exposed to an intact male while nursing, she can get pregnant again. The timing is such that about the same time her kittens are able to eat on their own, she can produce another litter. A nursing queen can also be spayed, but it is preferable to wait until after her kittens are weaned and her mammary glands are less engorged. By waiting, surgery time and blood loss are reduced, and the kittens will not require bottle feeding.

Q *What can be done to stop an accidental pregnancy?*

A At this time there are no drugs available that guarantee the safe termination of an unwanted pregnancy. Hormonal treatments and the drug prostaglandins are possible therapies, but there are risks, including sterilization, bone marrow suppression, mammary cancer, and diabetes. There are no safe birth control options that can be recommended for cats either, although progesterone containing compounds are sometimes used. The safest option for a cat who becomes pregnant is to complete the pregnancy or be sterilized and terminate the pregnancy. Intact females should be kept indoors and isolated from any intact males unless you want them to breed.

Q *At what age should I wean my kitten?*

A The weaning process naturally begins when kittens are about four weeks old. This is when they start developing their baby teeth and can start to eat solid food. Up until this time, kittens nurse from their mother or are bottle fed cat milk replacer. It becomes more difficult for the queen to produce enough milk to satisfy the hunger of multiple large kittens after four weeks.

There are various strategies for weaning kittens, and kittens can be introduced to canned kitten food, baby food, soaked and mashed dry kitten food, or human baby rice cereal as their first food. When kittens are first introduced to solid food, it is best to place it in a shallow plate to provide easy access. The weaning process is a dirty time for kittens, because they tend to walk through their food and get it all over themselves; have some kitten shampoo and cleaning supplies on hand. Kittens can be fully weaned by the time they are six weeks old. If a six-week-old kitten is still nursing, he should be separated from the queen for most of the day to encourage eating. This will also start the queen's "drying up" process, since the stimulation of nursing continues milk production.

Q *My male cat only has one testicle. Should I be concerned?*

A Testicles in a fetus start out in the abdominal cavity, but during development in utero, they migrate into the scrotum. Male cats are normally born with both testes descended into their scrotums. Some cats are born without fully descended testicles, and if they are not descended by four to six months of age, it is unlikely that they are going to pass into the normal location. When only one testicle is present in the scrotum, the condition is called cryptorchid. If a cat does not have any testicles in his scrotum, he is bilaterally cryptorchid. Retained testicles do not present a health risk.

Cryptorchid cats should still be neutered because their retained testicle still produce testosterone. A retained testicle can be found anywhere along the normal route that it would have descended—from the abdominal cavity to the inguinal ring to under the skin near the pubis or scrotum. Neutering a cryptorchid cat is more involved than a routine neuter because additional incisions and a probing of the abdominal cavity may be needed to locate the retained testicle.

Q What should I do about my cat's vaginal discharge?

A A veterinarian should examine any cat with a vaginal discharge as female cats should not normally have discharge from their vaginas. The age of your cat factors into what the discharge represents. Kittens can develop vaginitis, which appears as a milky, yellow discharge. A vaginal discharge in a pregnant cat who is not ready to queen can be a sign of infection or abortion. After queening, cats may have a bloody or dark discharge for a week. Vaginal discharges in mature female cats can be a sign of different stages of uterine infections—from milder metritis to life threatening pyometra.

To determine the cause of the discharge, your veterinarian takes a swab of the material to examine microscopically and see what kinds of cells are present. If the vet finds an infection, he or she will send the material to a lab for culture to determine what type of bacteria is present. X rays and ultrasound are other tests that can aid in diagnosing the problem. Whatever the means of discovery, once your vet has determined the cause he or she can prescribe a treatment.

Q Should I be concerned about a lump in my cat's mammary region?

A Your veterinarian should investigate any lumps or bumps on a cat, but those in the mammary region are of particular concern. Both males and females have nipples, usually four on each side, and can develop mammary cancer. The likelihood of mammary cancer in a female cat spayed before she reached puberty or in a male is slim. Intact females or those females who were spayed after starting their first heat cycle have a greater chance of contracting mammary cancer.

Both benign and malignant growths can occur in the mammary region. Benign growths can appear as cysts or present themselves during pregnancy or nursing when mammary glands are enlarged. The most common malignant growth is mammary tubular adenocarcinoma.

Benign growths tend to be soft and fluctuant, while malignant growths are more firm and solid. A veterinarian should examine any unknown mammary growth and perform a needle aspirate and/or biopsy to determine what is present.

Q *Is there anything I can do to help control the stray cat population?*

A Unfortunately, the stray cat population in the United States is out of control, but there are ways that concerned cat lovers can help. Most locales have rescue groups or other humane organizations that help to trap, sterilize, and release stray cats. The programs help stop the uncontrolled reproduction and allow the cats to live in stable feral colonies. Volunteering your time with one of these groups and/or giving them monetary donations is valuable.

Educate friends and neighbors about the importance of sterilizing cats, even if they are kept indoors. No one should be accidentally contributing to the cat overpopulation. Although research is currently underway to develop long-term oral sterilization for cats, this technology is not yet available. Until a vaccine is readily available, you can contact local animal rescue groups to see if they can help you trap and sterilize these cats.

Q *Is herpes transferable from a mother cat to her kittens?*

A Herpes conjunctivitis is common in cats. Kittens can be exposed to the virus from their mother if she has an active infection. Feline herpes is only transmissible between cats. Although the feline rhinotracheitis-calici-panleukopenia vaccine that all cats should receive protects against rhinotracheitis, another name for feline herpes, it decreases the associated clinical signs but does not prevent infection.

Aside from conjunctivitis, inflammation of the tissues around the eye, herpes can cause sneezing, nasal congestion, and excessive tearing. It is uncommon for cats to become blind from herpes, but scarring and corneal ulceration sometimes occurs in uncontrolled infections.

Q *I am interested in breeding my cat, but I am concerned about hip dysplasia. Is it hereditary?*

A Hip dysplasia is an abnormal conformation of the ball and socket hip joint. Most cats with hip dysplasia do not exhibit clinical signs, but those that do can show stiffness, crouching gait, lameness, an inability to jump, and pain.

How this defect is passed genetically is not clearly known. The condition is seen most frequently in Maine Coons, Persians, and Siamese cats. These cats are among the most popular breeds.

The feline prognosis is much better than that in dogs, due to differences in lifestyle and size. Medical treatment for the condition is aimed at reducing the inflammation and pain associated with arthritis and abnormal friction in the hip joints. In severe cases, a surgical procedure called a femoral head osteotomy is performed.

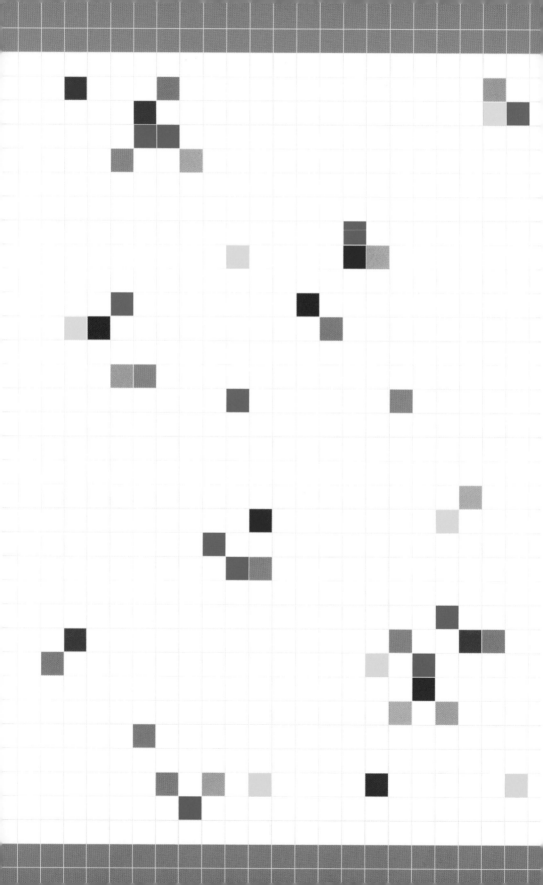

CHAPTER 7

Geriatrics

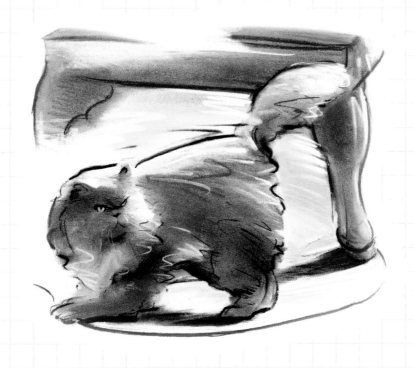

Getting old is never easy, and it is especially difficult for a cat who can't verbalize her aches and pains. The aging process will no doubt take a toll on your companion, but with some extra love and care, older cats can still live full lives and contribute much joy in their final years in your home. Knowing what to expect as your cat's body changes helps you to provide her the proper care and comfort to ensure a healthy quality of life in her later years.

Q How do I calculate the age of my cat in human years? When is a cat old?

A To calculate the age of your cat in human years, use the following guidelines. The first year of your cat's life is equal to about sixteen years in your life—cats go through birth to puberty to early adulthood all within a year. During the next two years she will mature the equivalent of six human years, and after that, each year is equal to four of ours. This means that twenty years in a cat's life corresponds to ninety-six years of human life. These guidelines relate to average cat aging and most cats live to be thirteen to fifteen years old (sixty-eight to seventy-six human years).

Veterinarians generally consider cats to be seniors at about nine years old, and most cats show measurable signs of aging by the time they are twelve years old. Health care for senior cats requires a lot of attention since every part of the body is affected by aging and certain diseases affect older cats more frequently. Some veterinarians offer senior health plans that monitor older cats for changes and detect problems at early stages, when they are most treatable. These plans can include blood tests, urinalysis, blood pressure measurement, and physical exams twice a year.

Q When is my cat too old to handle anesthesia?

A Age is never a reason to decline anesthesia. The decision to anesthetize your cat should be based on her health and medical condition. Examination and preanesthetic blood work determine the risks of anesthesia. A variety of fast-acting and safe injectable and inhalant anesthetic drugs makes tailoring anesthesia for specific situations possible. Extra precautions such as an IV catheter, fluids, reversal agents, and additional vital sign monitoring are also available to aid in adjusting anesthesia to individual conditions. If a veterinarian tells you not to perform a procedure due to the risk of anesthesia, seek out another opinion. A procedure such as extraction of an abscessed tooth performed under anesthesia removes infection and stops the pain your cat is experiencing. Ongoing pain and infection are more likely to shorten your cat's life than the anesthesia.

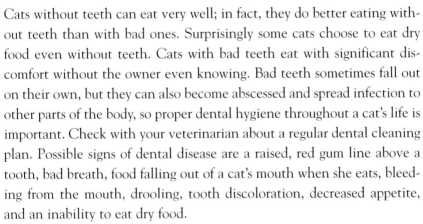

Q *Can my cat eat if she is missing teeth?*

A Cats without teeth can eat very well; in fact, they do better eating without teeth than with bad ones. Surprisingly some cats choose to eat dry food even without teeth. Cats with bad teeth eat with significant discomfort without the owner even knowing. Bad teeth sometimes fall out on their own, but they can also become abscessed and spread infection to other parts of the body, so proper dental hygiene throughout a cat's life is important. Check with your veterinarian about a regular dental cleaning plan. Possible signs of dental disease are a raised, red gum line above a tooth, bad breath, food falling out of a cat's mouth when she eats, bleeding from the mouth, drooling, tooth discoloration, decreased appetite, and an inability to eat dry food.

Dental health should be a concern throughout your cat's life, and regular dentistry helps to preserve teeth. Dentistry can be safely performed on geriatric cats with preanesthetic testing, proper anesthesia, and monitoring. Most problem cat teeth cannot be salvaged. Teeth that are broken, eroded, contain advanced cervical neck lesions, or have infected roots should be extracted as antibiotics are only a temporary measure against infection. After extraction, a soft diet, antibiotics, and pain relievers allow the gums to heal. Most owners admit that they did not realize how bad the dental problems were in their cat until they were treated and the owners saw the great response from their cat.

Q *What does it mean if my cat drinks excessive amounts of water?*

A Drinking excessively (more than about a cup of water a day) is called polydipsia. It can be a sign of disease or a response to environmental conditions and diet. For example, the latter can mean cats who eat exclusively dry food drink more than those who eat canned because canned food contains mostly water. Some cats drink an excessive amount of water for attention or because they like the taste of fresh water flowing out of a spigot. Generally, though, cats are not big water drinkers.

If your cat increases her water consumption, she should be examined and undergo a urinalysis. A urinalysis will reveal if the cat's kidneys are properly functioning, if infection of the urinary tract is present, or whether or not the cat has diabetes mellitus. A blood test gives additional information on these conditions.

Increased water consumption, increased urination, and weight loss are all signs typically found in cats with kidney disease or diabetes mellitus. Cats who drink a lot and are dehydrated should have concentrated urine with a low water content because the animal's body naturally tries to conserve water and balance hydration. Dehydrated cats with dilute urine are in trouble. Kidney disease and diabetes are both manageable but not curable conditions, depending upon the stages they are diagnosed.

Q *Can cats have high blood pressure?*

A Hypertension is the medical term for high blood pressure, and cats can have it. Veterinarians have been routinely measuring blood pressure in cats for only the past ten years or so because previously, none of the available devices gave accurate measurements. To get a reliable reading, a cat must remain calm, which is always a challenge in a veterinary clinic. Blood pressure values tend to start higher and come down when the cat's stress level decreases—some cats will not relax enough even for readings to be taken.

Feline hypertension can be primary, occurring on its own, or secondary to kidney disease or hyperthyroidism. Signs of hypertension include restlessness, increased vocalization, seizures, and other behavior changes. Cats with hypertension can suddenly go blind because of secondary retinal detachment, but controlling blood pressure often will allow the retina to reattach. Hypertension is managed with medications.

Q *What happens to a cat with hyperthyroidism?*

A Hyperthyroid cats produce too much T4, the active hormonal product of the thyroid gland. Thyroid hormone does not have one specific function but it interacts with other hormones and organs to regulate general metabolism. When cats have excessive levels of T4, they tend to have increased heart rates, act more restless and hyper, and lose weight. They usually have good or increased appetites and occasionally experience vomiting or diarrhea. Uncontrolled thyroid disease leads to high blood pressure (hypertension) and heart disease.

Hyperthyroidism is typically found in cats nine years and older. Your veterinarian can diagnose the disease through a blood test or a thyroid scan. Cats who have clinical signs consistent with the disease and normal T4 levels need to have an additional test called "T4 by equilibrium dialysis" performed. Hyperthyroidism is one of the most treatable and even curable diseases in older cats. There are three treatment options: long-term medication with methimazole given twice daily, surgical removal of the glands, or selective destruction of the overactive tissue with a special form of radiation called I-131. Cost, overall patient condition, ease of medicating, and owner preference are all factors in determining which treatment option to pursue.

Q *How can I tell if my cat has cancer?*

A Cancer is more common in cats eight years and older, but is not unheard of in younger cats. There are various forms of cancer—some are internal and some are external. External forms are much easier for you to find because you can feel or observe them during regular interaction with your cat. The signs of internal cancer are subtler. Although technology has advanced in veterinary medicine, specific blood tests for tumor markers are not yet available. Diagnosis is usually based on a physical exam, blood tests, X rays, ultrasound, endoscopy, and biopsy.

The development of lumps and bumps as your cat ages is not normal, so a veterinarian should check out any external growths you find. White cats or cats with white patches and pink noses are more at risk for squamous cell carcinoma, a type of skin cancer, because of the sun. Even if these types of cats are indoor cats, they are at risk because UV rays still come through the window. Intact female cats and cats spayed as adults have a higher chance of developing mammary tumors. Cats with cancer of internal organs show nonspecific signs, depending on the organs affected. Vomiting, diarrhea, anemia, weight loss, anorexia, dehydration, difficulty breathing, and weakness are all possible signs.

When cancer is diagnosed at an early stage, more treatment options are usually available. Options are based on the type of cancer and its location and may include surgery, chemotherapy, radiation, immunotherapy, cryotherapy, and laser therapy. You should discuss these options with your veterinarian. The prognosis for cats with cancer is variable, but with proper treatment, many cats can enjoy a good quality of life for an extended period or in some instances be cured.

Q Do cats get arthritis?

A Any animal can develop arthritis. Veterinarians call this condition degenerative joint disease (DJD). Cats may develop arthritis due to body shape, genetics, traumas they've experienced, and normal aging, which produces extra friction between the bones. DJD is a progressive disease in which extra calcification forms at sites of the increased friction within the joints, limiting the range of motion and putting strain on nearby tendons, ligaments, and nerves.

X rays are needed to definitively diagnose DJD and differentiate it from muscle weakness and spinal cord or nerve problems. Helping cats with DJD involves making their access to food, water, litter box, and sleeping areas easy. Some owners build steps or provide stools to give their cats easier access to favorite beds or resting areas. DJD is managed, not cured. Its progression can be slowed and the associated pain treated. The less a cat has to jump up or down, the slower DJD will progress. Various options for pain relief include low dose aspirin and corticosteroid drugs. Supplements containing glucosamine and chondroitin sulfate safely help many animals with DJD by improving the cartilage and fluid in joints, thus reducing painful friction.

Q How is heart disease diagnosed in cats?

A Heart disease is diagnosed through a combination of examination, heart auscultation (listening to the heart with a stethoscope), X ray, electrocardiogram (otherwise known as EKG), and ultrasound. Some cats are born with bad hearts and others develop heart disease due to a genetic predisposition or as a result of another disease. Unfortunately, some forms of heart disease are difficult to diagnose and may be apparent only when the cat's heart starts failing. Possible signs of heart disease are coughing, restlessness, open mouth breathing, weight loss, and general malaise.

Heart murmurs and arrhythmias are warning flags for heart disease. Not every cat with a murmur develops heart disease, but if a murmur is heard during an examination, the safest thing to do is follow up with X rays and an ultrasound. X rays show the size and shape of the heart and whether there is any secondary congestion in the lungs. Ultrasound allows examination of each heart chamber, muscle wall, and valve. It also shows how the blood is flowing and where turbulence is present.

Heart disease caused by hypertension, hyperthyroidism, or metabolic imbalance has the potential for cure or at least long-term management. The prognosis for cats with cardiomyopathy, heart muscle disease, is not as good. Treatment for these cats focuses on stimulating the heart to pump efficiently and decreasing the fluid loads it must handle. Unfortunately, once clinical signs of cardiomyopathy begin, the prognosis declines.

Q *How do I know when it is time to put my cat to sleep?*

A Ending a pet's life is one of the hardest decisions you will face during your lifetime. The decision is an individual one and should be based on the quality of life the cat is experiencing. Cats have a strong will to survive, so when they give up trying, it makes the decision easier. Most cats do not die peacefully just from old age. Instead they develop diseases or degenerate to the point where they can no longer maintain themselves, and they waste away. This is very difficult to watch, especially when the cat has been like a member of the family for many years.

Owners want to know when their cat is in pain, but that is a hard judgment call. Most of the life-ending conditions that develop do not cause pain, but they do cause nausea, exhaustion, and general discomfort—it is rare for a cat to cry out or moan in pain. I advise owners to assess how much the cat's behavior has changed: Does your cat want or have the ability to eat? Drink? Will she get up and use the litter box? Can she get around on her own? Does she respond to you? Consider the answers to these questions when making your decision.

Euthanasia is a personal decision, but it should be done because of love for the pet and the desire to end a downward spiral of discomfort. When a cat is "put to sleep," she is usually given an intravenous injection of pentobarbital—an overdose of an anesthetic agent. All of the muscles in the body relax, and the heart stops beating. As long as the vein being injected does not collapse, death comes within thirty seconds. You need to decide whether you want to be with your pet during the injection and how you want the remains handled. Private cremation or pet cemetery burial are two of the options.

Q *My cat has diabetes mellitus. What care do I need to provide her?*

A Like humans, cats can develop diabetes, a condition in which the body cannot utilize the sugar in the blood. The symptoms are similar to those of humans—increased thirst, increased urination, increased appetite with weight loss. Sometimes, your cat's pancreas cannot produce enough insulin to control his blood sugar level. This is called insulin-dependent diabetes. Conversely, the pancreas may produce insulin but the body does not respond to it. Either way, your cat will need to have special medical attention to regulate the condition. There are some things you can do to help prevent the onset of diabetes in your cat.

Try to feed your cat a high-quality, healthy diet. Obese cats are more susceptible to diabetes, so keep your cat's weight under control. Older cats are at risk for disease in general, so pay attention to changes in behavior, like excessive drinking and urination.

If your cat is diagnosed with diabetes, she will likely need twice daily insulin injections and a diet change. Some cats' diabetes can be managed with diet and oral medications. Your veterinarian will teach you how to give your cat injections and monitor his response. Life threatening hypoglycemia is possible if insulin is not injected properly or if the cat's need for insulin changes, so owners must observe their diabetic cats closely.

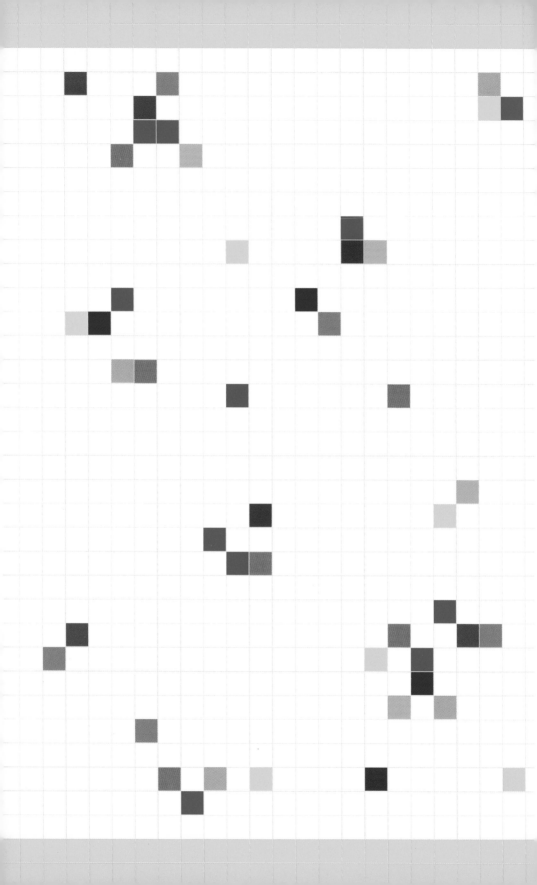

CHAPTER 8

General Health

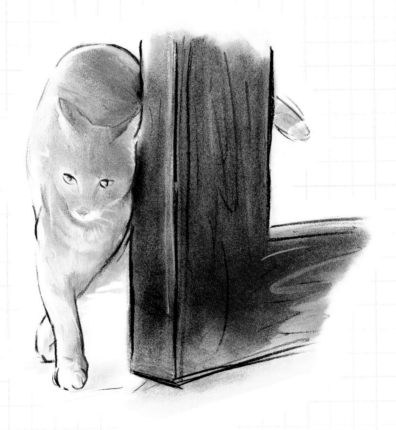

Everyone has basic questions about general cat care and health, but it is impossible to provide answers for each individual situation. The most commonly asked questions relate to breed, sex, and environment. The following are some of the most-asked questions from Cat Fancy readers.

Q What are some general ways I can help protect my cat from disease?

A To start, immunize your kitten. Kittens have immunity from their mothers after birth, but this maternal immunity wanes by twelve weeks of age. Subsequent immunity comes from vaccines and exposure to infectious agents, which creates antibodies. Not every cat needs every vaccine each year, so you should discuss your individual pet's needs with your veterinarian.

Feeding your cat a good quality diet that he enjoys and digests well is also necessary for maintaining health. Make sure you read the label of your cat's food because well-balanced cat foods that have passed the Association of American Feed Control Officials (AAFCO) feeding trials are guaranteed to provide adequate nutrition under normal conditions. Fresh, clean water should always be available.

Minimizing the stresses in your cat's life helps protect him against disease. Providing comfortable shelter and maintaining a clean litter box are two ways stress is minimized indoors. Outdoor stresses are harder to control because outdoor cats are exposed to parasites, other animals, and environmental conditions—all risks that can lead to disease.

Last but not least, pay attention to your cat. Recognizing changes in your cat's behavior and observing appetite, water consumption, and eliminations hopefully allows you to detect health problems at early stages.

Q Should I have my cat's teeth cleaned?

A Cats need a healthy mouth to survive because their eating, drinking, and grooming depends upon it. Dental health is influenced by genetics, diet, and home care. Preventive home care options include tooth brushing, oral rinses and wipes, and specially formulated treats and diets, but more serious conditions such as gingivitis require a visit to your veterinarian. Early signs of gingivitis include mouth odor and a red, raised line at the tooth-gum line. Without proper care, plaque and tartar build on the teeth and bacteria lodge within these substances, which damages the gums. Left untreated, tooth erosion, root infection, and penetration of bacteria into the sinuses or blood stream occur. Studies show that bad teeth are a source of infection that impacts other organs such as the kidneys, especially in geriatric cats.

To ensure a more serious condition does not occur, your cat's mouth needs to be examined at least annually by a veterinarian. During this exam your cat's gums, teeth, and tongue are evaluated for problems. If gingivitis, plaque, or tartar buildup is evident, the best treatment is a professional cleaning by your veterinarian. This process involves probing and evaluating each tooth, hand scaling, ultrasonic scaling, polishing, and a fluoride treatment while your cat is under general anesthesia. Although some cats may allow superficial scaling of their teeth, anesthesia is needed for a thorough procedure that uses sharp instruments under and around the gums. Diseased teeth are usually extracted. Some cats need annual or semiannual dental cleaning, while others require the procedure only once once or twice in a lifetime.

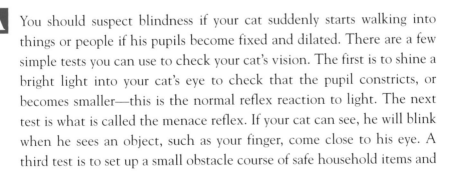

Q *How can I tell if my cat can't see?*

A You should suspect blindness if your cat suddenly starts walking into things or people if his pupils become fixed and dilated. There are a few simple tests you can use to check your cat's vision. The first is to shine a bright light into your cat's eye to check that the pupil constricts, or becomes smaller—this is the normal reflex reaction to light. The next test is what is called the menace reflex. If your cat can see, he will blink when he sees an object, such as your finger, come close to his eye. A third test is to set up a small obstacle course of safe household items and see if your cat easily maneuvers through it without bumping into things.

Blindness is not common in cats and development of complete cataracts is rare. As they age, cats develop a condition called lenticular sclerosis, which is a thickening and opacity of the lens, making it appear cloudy. Reduced night or dim light vision is normal in older cats. One cause of acute blindness in cats is high blood pressure. Hypertension causes retinal detachment, leading to a loss of vision. If detected and treated early, the retina can reattach and vision can be restored. Blindness is a condition warranting immediate veterinary attention.

Q What can I do if my cat's eye is red and squinting?

A A red, squinting eye is painful, so your cat may be reluctant to have you look at it. If you have saline eye drops available, you can attempt to flush the eye. However, a veterinarian should examine the cat to determine the specific cause. This often requires staining the eye, measuring tear production, applying a topical anesthetic so the eye can be better examined and the lids probed, and using an ophthalmoscope, or special lense, to look at deeper layers of the eye. Conjunctivitis, corneal ulcers, ocular foreign bodies, uveitis, and trauma are all possible causes. Once your veterinarian determines the cause, he or she can recommend appropriate treatment. Cats tend to rub an uncomfortable eye, which can potentially damage the eye further, so you may need to use a protective Elizabethan collar.

Q Can cats develop allergies?

A Cats can develop allergies and they can develop sensitivities to just about any substance in their environment including human dander. The most common sign of allergies in a cat is dermatitis, but your cat also may itch, lick excessively, or develop multiple small scabs (a condition called miliary dermatitis). Other signs of allergies in cats include sneezing, asthma, conjunctivitis, vomiting, and diarrhea.

It is often difficult to determine what triggers allergies in cats, but fleas are known to be the most common allergen. Allergy testing is available, and the method considered most accurate is intradermal skin testing. When an animal is skin tested, small amounts of potential allergens are injected under the skin, and the inflammatory reaction produced (a red, raised mark) is measured. The substances producing the most reaction are those to which the cat is most allergic. An alternative testing method involves measuring specific inflammatory antibody levels in the blood. The higher the level of antibody, the more allergic the animal is to the substance. To determine the presence of a food allergy, a hypoallergenic diet is fed exclusively to a cat for six to eight weeks. If the signs of allergy are relieved, then the veterinarian can confirm a diagnosis.

Allergies are generally managed rather than cured, and you can try a treatment involving medication with antihistamines or cortisone. If specific allergens are identified in testing, hyposensitization—desensitizing the cat to a small amount of antigens—with allergy shots is another option. More importantly, you should remove the irritating substance from your cat's environment whenever possible.

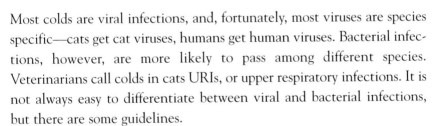

Q Can I catch a cold from my cat?

A Most colds are viral infections, and, fortunately, most viruses are species specific—cats get cat viruses, humans get human viruses. Bacterial infections, however, are more likely to pass among different species. Veterinarians call colds in cats URIs, or upper respiratory infections. It is not always easy to differentiate between viral and bacterial infections, but there are some guidelines.

Characteristics of viral URIs are clear discharges from the nasal area or eye, sneezing, and a fever that comes and goes. Cats usually continue to eat but are not as active. Cats with bacterial URIs tend to have persistent fevers, enlarged lymph nodes, green to yellow eye or nasal discharge, lethargy, and loss of their appetite. Cats' symptoms are very much like human common cold symptoms.

Treatment for a viral infection involves maintaining hydration and nutrition and supporting the immune system. Bacterial infections require antibiotics. Regardless of the type of infection, owners should wash their hands and avoid touching their faces after handling a sick cat. This will also help prevent transmission to other cats in the household, if there are any. Isolating a sick cat from other cats in the household is usually not beneficial because all the cats were exposed to the same agents that caused the infection before the clinical signs developed.

Q What should I do if my cat is straining to urinate?

A Straining is one sign of a urinary blockage in a male cat—a potentially life threatening condition. First you should check to see if your cat is passing urine. Cats only slightly differ their postures when urinating and defecating so owners easily confuse constipated cats with those straining to urinate. If a male cat is straining and not passing urine, a veterinarian should examine him immediately. Straining occurs when infection or irritating materials inflame a cat's bladder or urethra. If you notice your cat straining and blood is present in the urine, this is a sign of lower urinary tract disease (LUTD). Regardless of the cause of straining, your cat is in discomfort and should receive medical attention.

After an examination to determine if a blockage is present, a veterinarian will perform a urinalysis. This test shows whether bacteria, crystals, or inflammation are responsible for the straining. Bacterial infections are actually the least common of the three. There are different types of crystals and stones that can develop in the urinary tract and cause blockage or irritation. Diet has a large impact on crystal formation within the urine. Canned diets are better for cats who develop crystals or benign bladder inflammation because they lead to the production of larger volumes of more dilute urine that flushes the bladder. The decision to feed a cat a diet specially formulated for urinary tract disease should be made after consulting your veterinarian. Do not feed a cat any special diet without consulting an expert.

Inflammation without crystals or bacteria can also cause straining. A benign, inflammatory condition of the bladder, called interstitial cystitis, occurs in some cats. Stress can trigger this condition, but most often a specific cause is not identified.

If a cat has recurrent bouts of LUTD or straining, further tests such as a urine culture, X ray, or ultrasound are needed to determine the cause. Specific management of the condition is based on the cause but may include special diet and medications that relieve pain and calm the lining of the bladder.

Q What should I do if my cat gags and wheezes?

A A cat with respiratory disease looks like he is gagging on a hairball but produces nothing when he gags. Gagging progresses to wheezing, and if left untreated, it can progress further to open mouth breathing and distress. These signs warrant a trip to the veterinarian, who should proceed to examine your cat and take chest X rays. Without X rays, it is impossible to determine what is going on. Any disease of the heart or lungs potentially causes gagging or difficulty with breathing.

A common cause of gagging and wheezing is feline asthma. Allergies or irritants trigger the airways (bronchi) to swell and become full of secretions during an asthma attack. This is dangerous because it limits the amount of oxygen that can pass through your cat's lungs. Prompt treatment with bronchodilators and cortisone (for anti-inflammatory effects) is needed for asthmatic cats, and those in more severe respiratory distress require oxygen. Other treatments for asthmatic cats include the human asthma drug, Accolate and the antihistamine, cyproheptadine. Human inhalers are useful in managing feline asthma and decrease the need for long-term internal cortisone with its side effects. Special chambers (tubes with valves that hold the aerosol) are needed to deliver inhaler drugs to cats since it is difficult to make them breath in at the correct time. Your veterinarian will know the best solution to treat your cat's wheezing and gagging.

Potential household triggers of asthma are cigarette or cigar smoke, construction, new carpeting, and even certain types of kitty litter. Stress also exacerbates asthma. Some asthma is due to seasonal allergies, even in indoor cats, but others are affected chronically due to environmental allergens present at all times.

Q *My cat's coat doesn't look good. Could there be a problem?*

A The condition of a cat's coat is determined by many different factors—genetics, diet, fleas or other parasites, self grooming, and general health. Long-haired cats, such as Persians, have hair that easily mats. Breeds such as the sphinx have greasy skin. Cats eating a poor-quality diet lose hair and have sticky coats. Cats with fleas are dirty and if they scratch excessively will have areas with sores and hair loss. Overweight cats cannot reach and groom themselves normally. They tend to get greasy and scaly along their backs, and the area under their tails becomes soiled. Cats with intestinal disease and malabsorption of nutrients have dry, dull coats.

The skin is the largest organ of your cat's body, and it reflects the general health of your cat. A change in the texture and appearance of the skin and coat can indicate internal health problems. Monitoring a cat's coat is part of the routine health care regimen, and your veterinarian should examine any noticeable changes, make care recommendations, and perform diagnostic testing if disease is suspected.

Q *I would like to take my cat on vacation with me. What steps should I take to prepare him for a trip?*

A Cats aren't natural travelers the way that dogs are, but they can enjoy the trip if you prepare them. Make an appointment with your veterinarian prior to travel to assure that your cat's vaccinations are up-to-date and that he is healthy enough to make a trip. If you will be traveling on a plane, you will need to have a health certificate from your vet. Discuss the ramifications of air travel with your vet, as some animals may not be suited to the special conditions like pressurized air or sudden temperature changes if your pet will be traveling as cargo. If you plan ahead with the airline, you may be able to keep your cat in the passenger cabin as long as he remains within a carrier that meets airline specifications. Discuss your cat's disposition with your vet as well. If, for example, your cat is easily agitated by a 15 minute car ride, he may not be the best candidate for a four hour plane ride. Your vet can also discuss the possibility of sedation, which may make the trip more comfortable for both you and your cat.

Prior to travel, whether by car or air, purchase a quality pet carrier. Check with your airline for a list of approved carriers. Durability is especially important if your cat will travel on a plane as cargo, as he could be jostled during the loading process. The carrier should be roomy enough for your cat to comfortably lie down and turn around. If your cat will travel with you in the cabin or on a road trip in the car, you can also consider a soft-sided carrier. Other important items for travel include: food and water with bowls or collapsible containers, first-aid supplies, medications, toys, litter box and litter, your cat's identification, and an appropriate restraining device.

 ## Should I get pet insurance?

It is worth investigating pet insurance for your cat. There are only a couple of companies that provide pet health insurance, and there are various levels of policy coverage. Even if you have insurance, you will be required to pay for veterinary services when they are provided, and then submit a claim to the insurance company who will then reimburse you directly for the covered amount.

Many policies do not cover pre-existing health conditions, and most policies pay only a percentage of the veterinary fees. Although insurance is useful for most cats, cats that go outdoors are at more risk for trauma, injury, and exposure to disease, so would likely benefit the most from coverage. Premiums are affordable for most pet owners.

Q *My cat is shaking his head and scratching his ears. What, besides ear mites, can cause this?*

A Your cat may have a bacterial or yeast infection of the ear, excessive wax buidup, allergies, or he may even have a polyp within his ear canal. These diagnoses are distinguished by examination of the ear with an otoscope and analyzing the material within the ear canal. Microscopic examination and culture may be needed. Yeast infections can prove troublesome and recurrent.

There are ear drops that contain antifungal agents, antibiotics, and cortisone that relieve irritation and kill the infectious organisms. Regular ear cleaning with specially formulated low pH products can control bacteria and yeast as well as cut down on wax and moisture buildup. If polyps are present, surgical removal may be warranted.

Q *What can I do to prevent impacted anal glands?*

A Cats have glands inside their anuses, located at approximately 5 and 7 o'clock. These structures secrete a foul-smelling liquid to waxy material. Most cats express these glands when they defecate or when they get excited. Diet, activity level and weight all contribute to anal gland impaction. Overweight, inactive cats tend to experience more problems. Adding fiber to your cat's diet may help.

If your cat has recurrent problems, they can be permanently removed through surgery, but this is rarely necessary. Manual expression every few weeks can help. I find that filling the glands with antibiotic/cortisone ointment after an impaction often eliminates future problems.

Q *Should I worry if my cat pants excessively?*

A Most cats do not pant, and when they do, they should be checked for medical problems. Diseases of the heart and airways (nose to lungs) can affect blood oxygenation and circulation, triggering panting.

A physical exam with a careful review of the heart and lungs is the first step in working up panting, followed by chest X-rays. If the findings are normal, significant disease causing the panting is unlikely. An echocardiogram (ultrasound of the heart) is the best way to assess the function and condition of the heart, so performing this test will confirm a healthy or diseased heart. Hopefully the results will be normal and your cat is merely panting due to overexertion, excitement, or stress.

Q *How often should I take my cat to the veterinarian?*

A Your cat should have a routine physical examination performed by your veterinarian once a year, with more frequent visits if he has specific health problems. Your veterinarian will want to examine the cat's entire body and make notations of any significant changes, take his temperature, weigh him, and listen to his heart and lungs. Vaccines are given based on need and may not be required annually. The time you spend during an annual visit discussing your cat's lifestyle, nutritional needs, behavior, and health will do more to protect his health than any vaccine booster.

Q *How do I deal with the death of my cat?*

A Everyone deals with grief differently. Whether you had to put your cat to sleep or he died naturally, the loss is never easy.

Your grief is justified, so remember to take time to care for yourself. Share your feelings with family members, friends, or other cat lovers. You might choose to have a small family service, whether at a pet cemetery or in your own backyard. Remember, if you have children, they need to grieve too. Sometimes, the death of a pet is the first death experience for a child, so it is an opportunity for you to explain the process of dying.

Pet cemeteries and private cremation are special options for taking care of a pet's remains. Your veterinarian may have a list of reputable pet cemetaries, cremation services, hotlines or discussion groups that can provide emotional support if you need more help with reaching closure.

Conclusion

Cat ownership requires an emotional and financial commitment. Your cat relies on you to provide for his basic needs and in return your cat provides you, in his unique way, love and companionship. By taking an active role in your cat's overall health, you can help ensure your cat gets the care he needs. Just reading a book such as this one helps educate you on potential signs of problems that you may not have otherwise noticed.

It also helps to have a good relationship with a competent veterinarian. Regular health care includes an annual physical exam and any vaccinations deemed necessary, based on your cat's lifestyle. Even though your cat may not need an annual vaccination, the time you and your vet spend discussing your cat during the annual physical examination is beneficial to you cat's overall health. When choosing a veterinarian, base your decision on the following: a recommendation from a friend or neighbor; the veterinarian's specialty; the services that are provided at the clinic; and convenience—is the vet close to home or does the clinic have extended hours?

Some of the best traits that cats possess are stoicism and a strong will to live, but these also work to their detriment because it's difficult for their owners to detect problems. Cats are complex creatures with relatively simple needs. If you have a good understanding of your cat's basic care and health, you can ensure a long, healthy life for your cat.

Index

A

accidents, car, 58
age/aging
    anesthesia in older cats, 72–73
    arthritis, 76–77
    calculating cat years to human years, 72
    cancer, 75–76
    euthanasia, 78
    excessive drinking, 74
    heart disease, 77–78
    high blood pressure (hypertension), 74–75
    hyperthyroidism, 75
    missing teeth, 73
AIDS, 43
allergies, 84–85
anal glands, 59, 90
anesthesia, 72–73
Animal Poison Control Center, 19, 57
antifreeze, 56–57
arthritis, 76–77
asthma, 87–88

B

biting, 11
bladder problems, 86
bleeding, 55
blindness, 75, 83–84
broken bones, 56

C

calicivirus, 43
cancer, 49, 67–68, 75–76
cataracts (lenticular sclerosis), 83–84
cat scratch disease, 34–35
chewing, 11–12
Chlamydia, 46
claws, 10–11, 48, 55
coat condition, 88
colds, 85–86
colitis, 23, 59
collars, 48
constipation, 24–25, 59
cryptorchid, 66

D

dangers to cats
    antifreeze, 56–57
    aspirin, 53–54
    collars, 48
    eating prey, 26
    phosphates in enemas, 25
    playing with dangerous toys, 25–26
    swallowing of foreign objects, 25–26, 57–58
dangers to humans
    cat bites, 11
    cat scratch disease, 34–35
    colds, 85–86
    mange, 33
    parasites, 31
    pregnant women's dangers, 34
    rabies, 44-45
    ringworm, 33
death, 78
declawing, 48
defecation, 13–14, 24–25
degenerative joint disease (DJD), 76–77
dehydration, 74

dental health. See teeth/dental health

diabetes, 74, 79

diet/nutrition, 22–24, 27, 82, 88

digital tenotomy, 48

diseases/disorders. See also emergencies; medications; vaccines/vaccinations

  allergies, 36, 84–85

  arthritis, 76–77

  asthma, 87

  Bartonella henselae, 34–35

  Bordatella bronchiseptica, 47

  cancer, 67–68, 75–76

  Chlamydia, 46

  coccidia/Giardia, 31–32

  cryptorchid, 66

  diabetes, 74, 79

  eye problems, 84

  feline AIDS, 44

  feline calicivirus, 43

  feline herpesvirus (rhinotracheitis), 42–43

  feline immunodeficiency virus (FIV), 44, 47

  feline infectious peritonitis (FIP), 46

  feline leukemia virus (FeLV), 43–44

  feline panleukopenia virus, 43

  gagging/wheezing, 87–88

  gastrointestinal problems, 31–32

  Giardia lamblia, 47

  heart disease, 77–78

  heartworm, 35–36

  high blood pressure (hypertension), 74–75

  hypertension, 84

  hyperthyroidism, 75

  jaundice, 26–27

  kidney problems, 74

  lenticular sclerosis, 84

  Lyme disease, 35

  mange, 33

  preventing, 82

  rabies, 44–45

  ringworm, 33, 46–47

  toxoplasmosis, 34

  upper respiratory infections (URIs), 85

  urinary problems, 86–87

  uterine infections, 63

  vaginal discharge, 67

  worms, 30–31

  wounds, 54

E

ear mites, 37

eating, stopping, 22–23

emergencies

  antifreeze ingestion, 56–57

  broken bones, 56

  gagging/wheezing, 87

  ingested foreign bodies, 25–26

  jaundice, 26–27

  overheating, 55–56

  preventing/planning ahead for, 52

  straining to urinate, 86–87

euthanasia, 78

excessive drinking, 74

excessive grooming, 12–13

eye problems, 75, 83–84

F

fatty liver disease (hepatic lipidosis), 22

feline immunodeficiency virus (FIV), 44, 47

fevers, 52–54

fiber supplements, 24, 25, 59
fighting, 54
first aid. See diseases/disorders; emergencies; toxic substances
fleas/flea control, 31, 32, 33
food, 22, 23
fractures, 56
FRCP (feline rhinotracheitis, calici, panleukopenia) vaccine, 42–43
fungal infections, 33, 46–47
fur, 88

G
gagging/wheezing, 87–88
gastrointestinal problems, 31–32
gestation, 64–65
Giardia lamblia, 47
gingivitis, 83
grooming (by cat), excessive, 12–13
grooming (by owner), combing/brushing, 25
guidelines for vaccinations, 41–42, 46–47

H
hairballs, 12–13, 25, 59
hair condition, 88
heart disease, 77–78
heartworm disease, 35–36
heat cycles, 63
herbal remedies, 13, 14, 18
herpes conjunctivitis, 68
herpesvirus (rhinotracheitis), 43
hiding, 17
high blood pressure (hypertension), 74–75
hip dysplasia, 69
hormone therapy, 15, 16
hunting, 26
hypertension, 84

hyperthyroidism, 75

I
identification, 48–49
immunization, 82. See also vaccines/vaccinations
infectious peritonitis (FIP), 46
insect stings, 58
insurance, pet, 89
itching, 84–85

J
jaundice, 26–27

K
kidney problems, 74
kittens, 31, 47, 65–66, 67

L
laxatives, 24
lenticular sclerosis, 84
leukemia virus (FeLV), 42, 43–44
linear foreign bodies, 25–26, 57–58
litter boxes, 13, 33
liver problems, 22–23
lost cats, 48–49
lumps, 67–68, 76
Lyme disease, 35

M
mammary lumps, 67–68
mange, 33
medications. See also vaccines/vaccinations
    administering, 40–41
    antianxiety, 12, 13, 14–15, 16
    vaccinations, 41–43
meowing, 18–19
missing teeth, 73
mites, 33

N
neutering, 15, 54, 62–64
new cats, introducing, 16
nursing mothers, 65

O
Oriental Shorthair, 18
overheating, 55–56

P
panleukopenia virus, 43
parasites
    ear mites, 83–84
    toxoplasmosis, 34
    worms, 30–31
pheromones, 15
plants, eating of, 19
poisons, 57–58
pregnancy, 64–65

R
rabies, 44–45
regurgitation, 23
ringworm, 33, 46–47

S
scratching, furniture, 10–11
sedation, 18
senior cats. See age/aging
skin, 88
    allergies, 84–85
    mange, 33
    ringworm, 33, 46–47
spaying, 15, 62–65, 68
spraying, 13–15, 15–16, 64
sterilization, 62–64, 68
stings, insect, 58
stools, 23–24, 36–37, 59
straining to urinate, 86–87
stress, 17–18, 82

T
teeth/dental health, 22, 47, 73,
    82–83
temperature, normal/high, 52–53
territorial behavior, 15
testicles, 66
thyroid disease, 75
ticks, 35
toxic substances
    Animal Poison Control Center,
    57
    antifreeze, 56–57
toxoplasmosis, 34
travel, with pets, 88–89

U
upper respiratory infections (URIs),
    87
urine/urination, 13–15, 24, 26, 64,
    86–87
uterine infections, 63

V
vaccines/vaccinations, 31–43, 45,
    49, 53
vaginal discharge, 67
veterinarian visits, 17–18, 52, 89
    See also emergencies
vision, 75, 83–84
vomiting, 23

W
weaning kittens, 65–66
weight, healthy, 27
wheezing, 87–88
worms, 30–31
wounds, 54